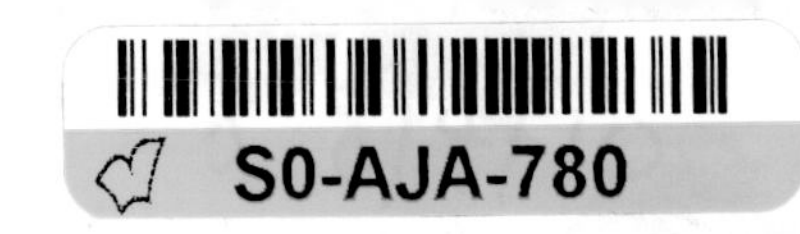

Dear David + Danielle,

Congrats on your marriage... now come on up to Sonoma County + explore.

Love You,

Dreamer

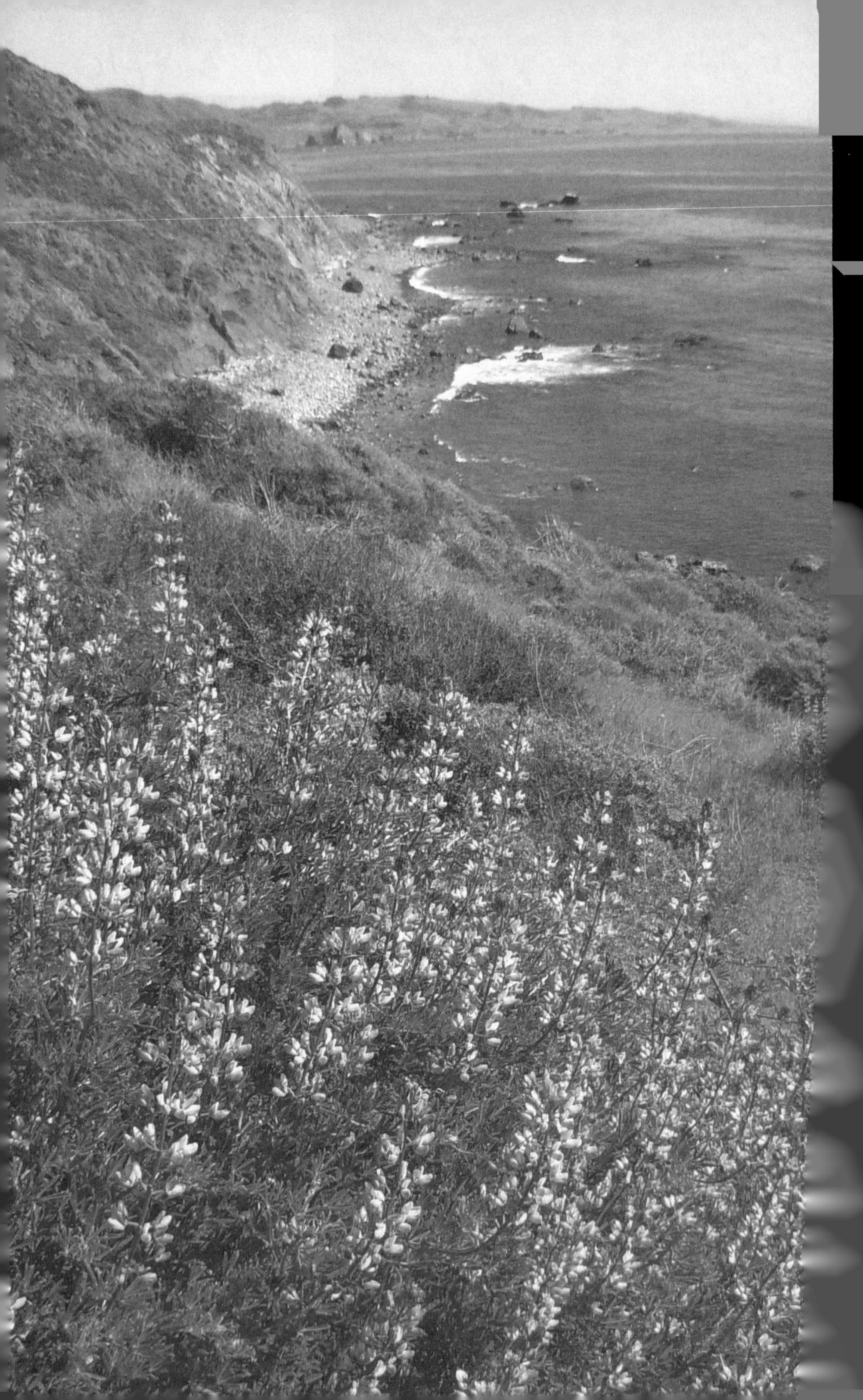

Hiking & Adventure Guide to the
Sonoma Coast & Russian River

Stephen W. Hinch

WILDERNESS PRESS . . . *on the trail since 1967*

BERKELEY, CA

Dedication

To Nicki, Greg, and Juliana

Hiking & Adventure Guide to the Sonoma Coast & Russian River

1st EDITION 2009

Interior photos, except where noted, by the author
Line illustrations by the author
Maps: Stephen W. Hinch
Cover design: Lisa Pletka and Scott McGrew
Book design and production: Larry B. Van Dyke

ISBN 978-0-89997-502-3

Manufactured in the United States of America

Published by: **Wilderness Press**
1345 8th Street
Berkeley, CA 94710
(800) 443-7227; FAX (510) 558-1696
info@wildernesspress.com
www.wildernesspress.com

Visit our website for a complete listing of our books and for ordering information.

Front cover photos: *(clockwise from top):* Goat Rock from Blind Beach; Rhododendrons at Kruse Rhododendron State Reserve; Cannon and Chapel at Fort Ross; Tafoni at Salt Point

Back cover photos: *(left to right):* Blind Beach Trail; Preparing the feast at Fort Ross Cultural Heritage Day; Lupine in bloom at Cardiac Hill

Frontispiece: Bush Lupine along Cardiac Hill Trail

SAFETY NOTICE: Although Wilderness Press and the author have made every attempt to ensure that the information in this book is accurate at press time, they are not responsible for any loss, damage, injury, or inconvenience that may occur to anyone while using this book. You are responsible for your own safety and health. The fact that an activity or a trail is described in this book does not mean that it will be safe for you. Be aware that trail conditions can change from day to day. Always check local conditions, know your own limitations, and consult a map.

Acknowledgments

It isn't possible to write a book like this without help from a lot of people. I first thank my wife, Nicki, who continues to provide unwavering support of my various writing projects. She not only gave excellent advice and proofread the manuscript, she also helped me map many of the trails.

Speaking of mapping trails, I would like to thank Lincoln Turner for accompanying me on some of the trips and for taking on the job of mapping the most challenging trail in the book, the East Austin Creek—Gilliam Creek Loop Trail. It was a worthy task for a person who, at an age when most of us begin to think about retiring, hiked the Grand Canyon from South Rim to North Rim *and back*, all in a 24-hour period while carrying a 40-lb pack! This was one of the trails he used to prepare for that adventure.

From California State Parks I would like to thank Jeremy Stinson, Heidi Horvitz, Jack Ekstrom, and Rick Royer for the information they provided as I prepared the chapters on state parks. And I would especially like to recognize Robin Joy Wellman for her excellent work above and beyond the call of duty in reviewing my chapter on Fort Ross. I also appreciate the encouragement I received from District Superintendent Liz Burko and Sector Superintendent Linda Rath.

From the Sonoma County Regional Parks, I appreciate the help provided by Steve Ehret and Ken Krout. A chance encounter with Ken in the field gave me valuable insight into the latest changes in these parks.

I would also like to recognize several other people whose assistance has made this a better book. Ruth Kirkpatrick taught me about ferns and helped identify specimens. Bea Brunn from the Stewards of the Coast and Redwoods provided excellent insight into the natural history of gray whales. Stewards Executive Director Michele Luna has also been a strong advocate of my work.

Finally, I would like to thank Roslyn Bullas of Wilderness Press for making this book a reality. She has been a pleasure to work with and provided tireless encouragement during the many long months I spent writing the manuscript.

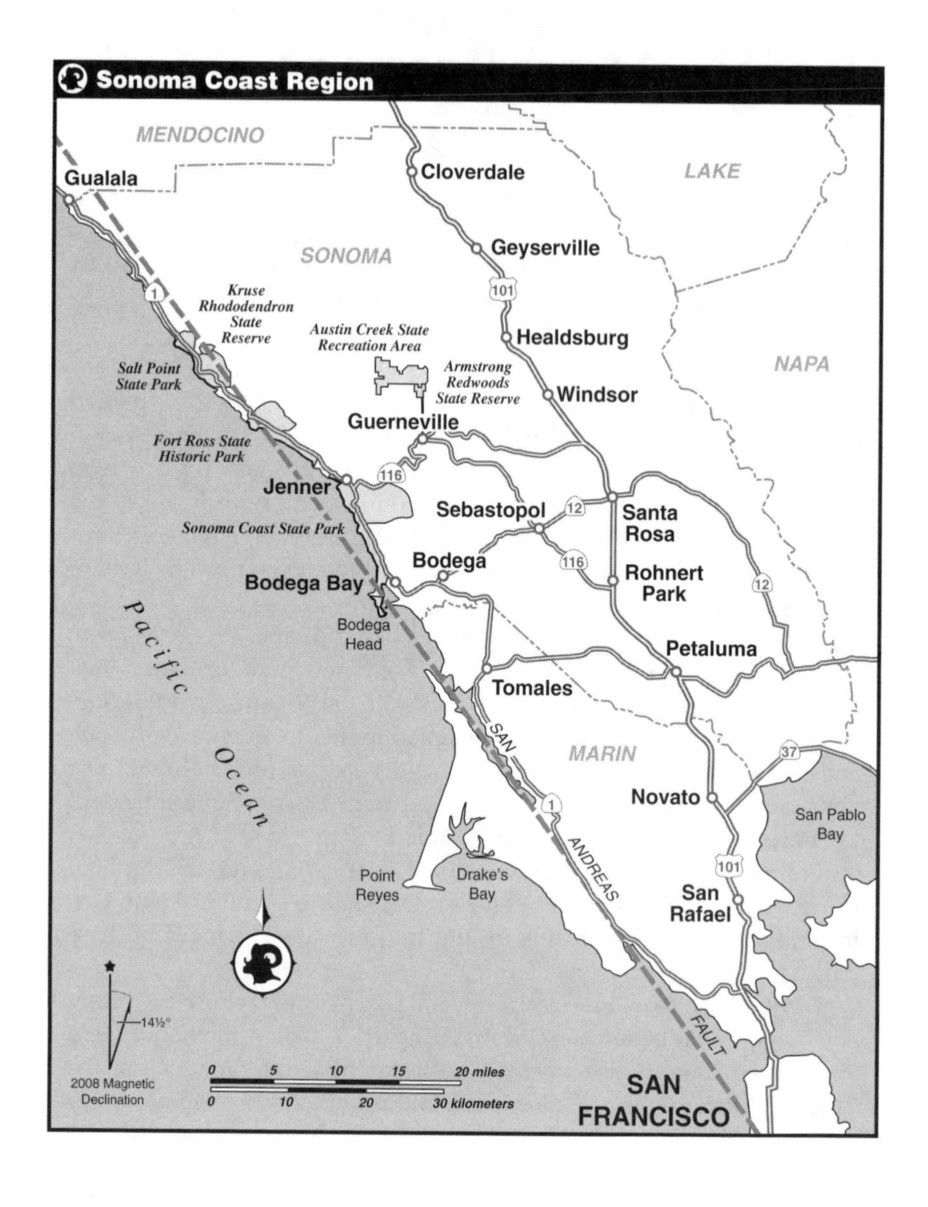

Sonoma Coast Region
MENDOCINO
LAKE
SONOMA
NAPA
MARIN
Gualala
Cloverdale
Geyserville
Healdsburg
Windsor
Guerneville
Jenner
Sebastopol
Santa Rosa
Bodega
Bodega Bay
Rohnert Park
Petaluma
Tomales
Novato
San Rafael
SAN FRANCISCO
Kruse Rhododendron State Reserve
Austin Creek State Recreation Area
Armstrong Redwoods State Reserve
Salt Point State Park
Fort Ross State Historic Park
Sonoma Coast State Park
Bodega Head
Point Reyes
Drake's Bay
San Pablo Bay
Pacific Ocean
SAN ANDREAS FAULT
1
101
116
12
37
14½°
2008 Magnetic Declination
0 5 10 15 20 miles
0 10 20 30 kilometers

Table of Contents

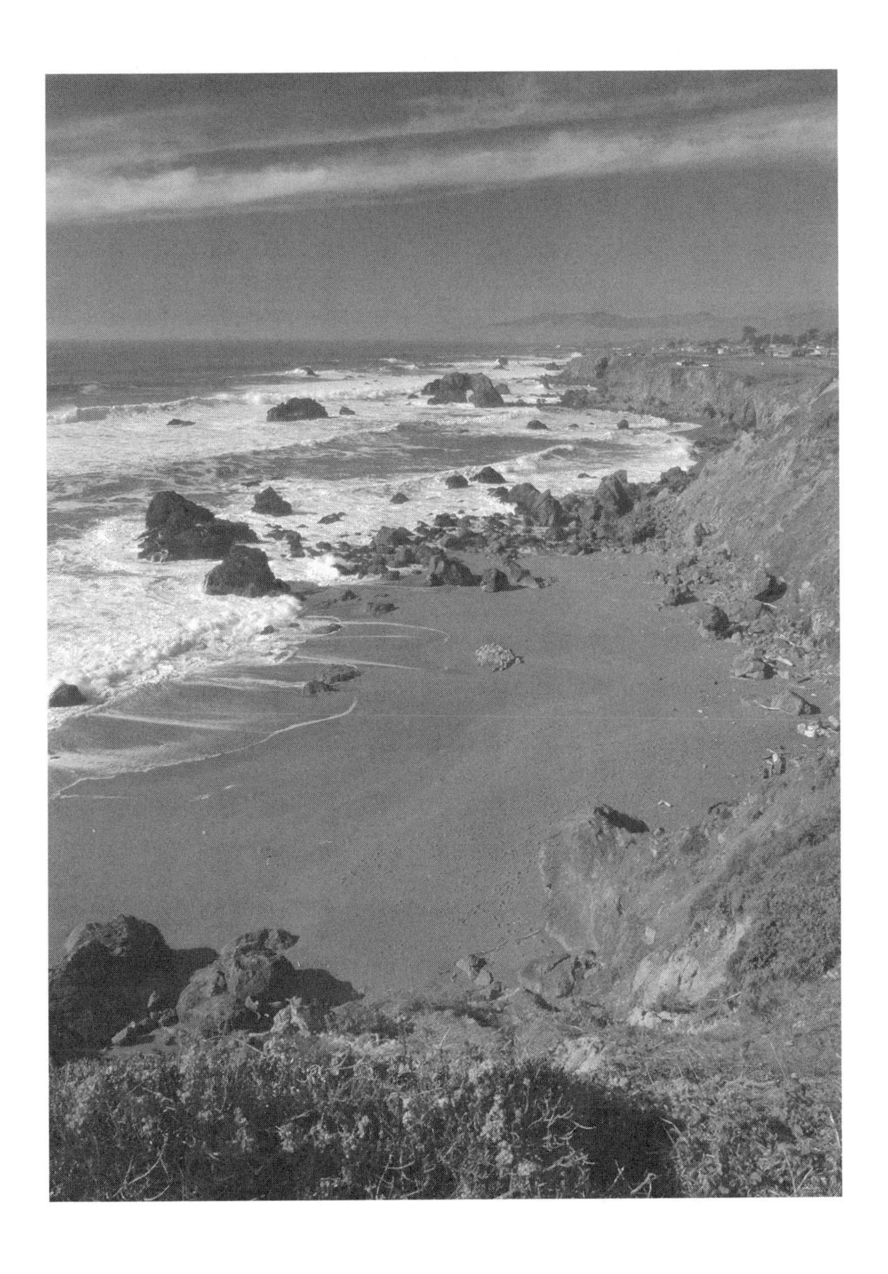

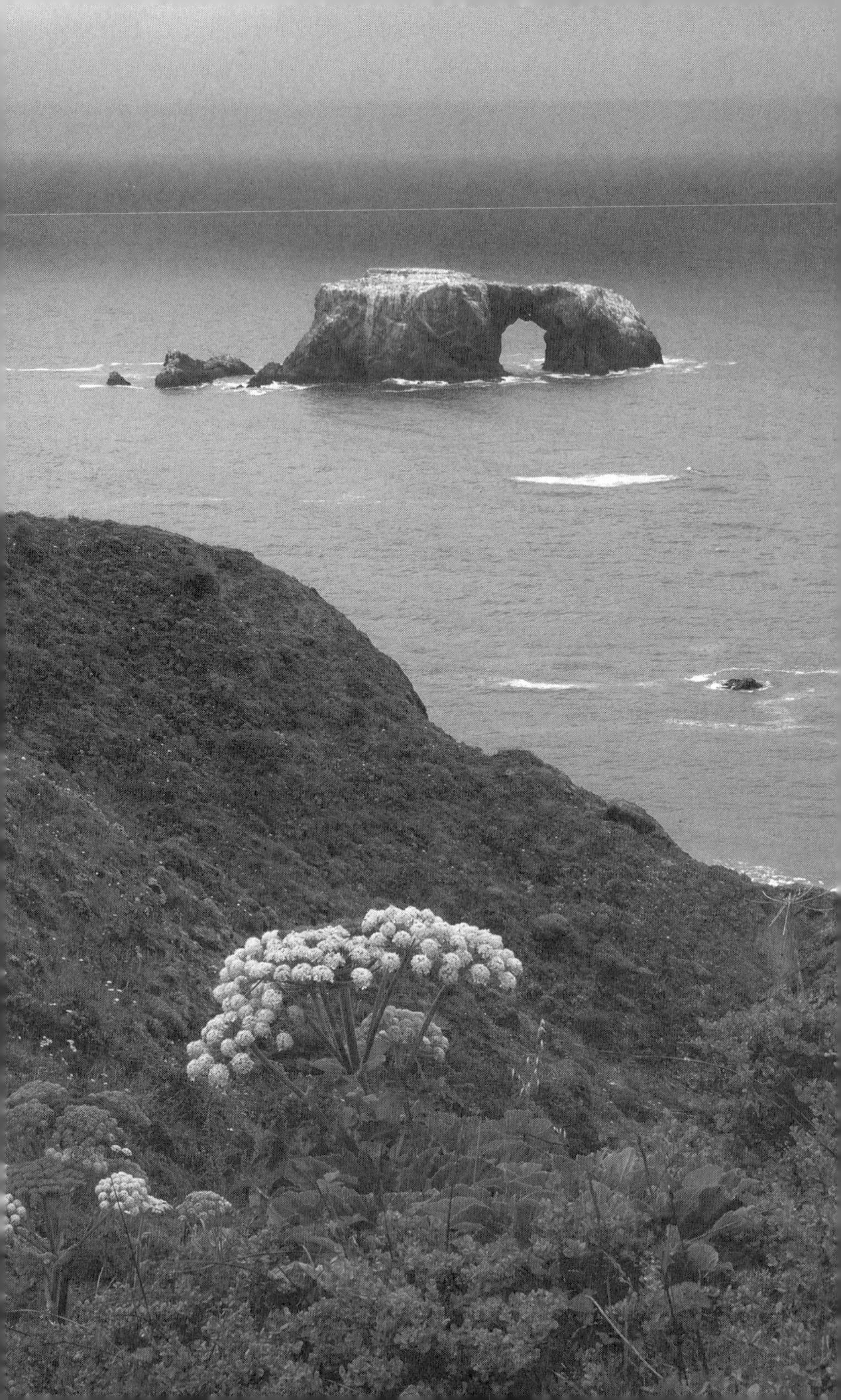

Chapter 1

Introduction to the Sonoma Coast

An hour's drive north of San Francisco lies one of the most spectacular sections of Pacific shoreline in all of California. Stretching from Bodega Bay to Gualala Point, the Sonoma Coast extends across 60 miles of windswept cliffs, isolated beaches, and crashing surf. Painters, photographers, and poets have all been inspired by Sonoma County's shores. Countless others have come to explore a surging tidepool or bask in the glow of a red Pacific sunset.

Four state parks help protect the natural beauty and historical significance of this magnificent coast, and two more lie a dozen miles inland. Sonoma Coast State Park, Fort Ross State Historic Park, Salt Point State Park, Kruse Rhododendron State Natural Reserve, Armstrong Redwoods State Natural Reserve, and Austin Creek State Recreation Area are all easily accessible and open to a wide range of pursuits.

Each park has a distinctive character. Sonoma Coast State Park is a geological wonder and is a popular escape from summer heat. At Fort Ross, the emphasis is on the history of a restored Russian stockade. Outdoor activities such as hiking, fishing, and abalone diving are the primary draw at Salt Point, while colorful rhododendron blooms bring throngs of visitors to Kruse Rhododendron State Reserve each spring. Armstrong Redwoods protects the last major stand of old-growth redwoods in Sonoma County, and nearby Austin Creek offers panoramic views from its oak-covered hillsides.

The County of Sonoma also hosts an extensive network of regional parks in the area—nine on the coast and seven more along the Russian River. Activities at these parks include camping, hiking, boating, fishing, swimming, birding, and picnicking, so there is something for everyone here.

The Sonoma Coast is a region of great geologic activity. Even the casual observer will notice the rugged nature of the shore, but if you really get out and explore, you'll find much more evidence of upheaval.

Left: *Arched Rock.*

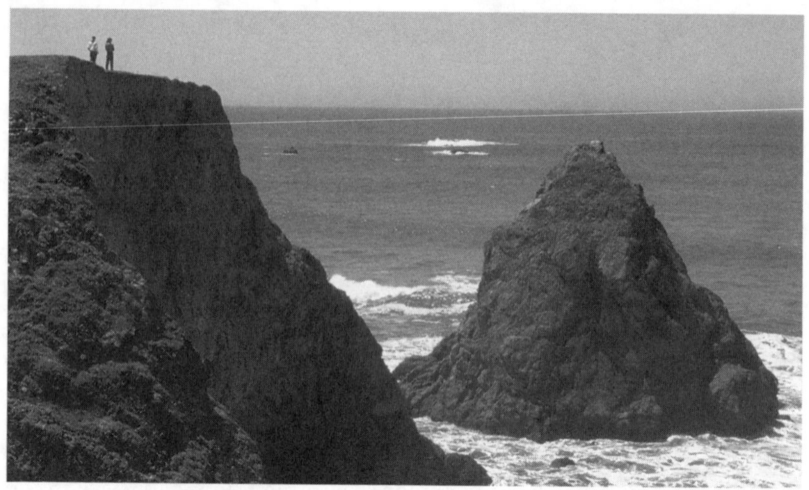

Hikers take in the view along the rugged Sonoma coastline.

In the hills above the coast, great rifts scar the earth. Elongated ponds of water stand incongruously atop ridges where no streams can fill them. Fences and roads jog abruptly, as if built by separate groups who couldn't agree on where to meet. To really understand this coast, we first need a brief lesson in geology.

A Land in Upheaval

Take a map of Sonoma County and study the shape of its coast. Start in the south at Bodega Head, a finger of land that juts into the sea on the west side of Bodega Bay. From here, follow the coastline south to Tomales Bay, a long, narrow inlet in Marin County that looks like, but isn't, the mouth of a large river.

Now take a ruler, draw a line through the middle of Tomales Bay, and continue northwestward into Sonoma County. The line will cut across Bodega Head, then run out to sea before making landfall again just south of Fort Ross. From there it will follow the South Fork of the Gualala River all the way into Mendocino County.

The line you have drawn is the great San Andreas Fault. Stretching for 800 miles from Southern California to the Mendocino Coast, the San Andreas is perhaps the most famous region of earthquake activity in the entire world. It was here near Tomales Bay (actually a fault valley long ago flooded by the sea) where the earth ruptured to cause the great San Francisco earthquake of 1906. The fault moved again in 1989 near San

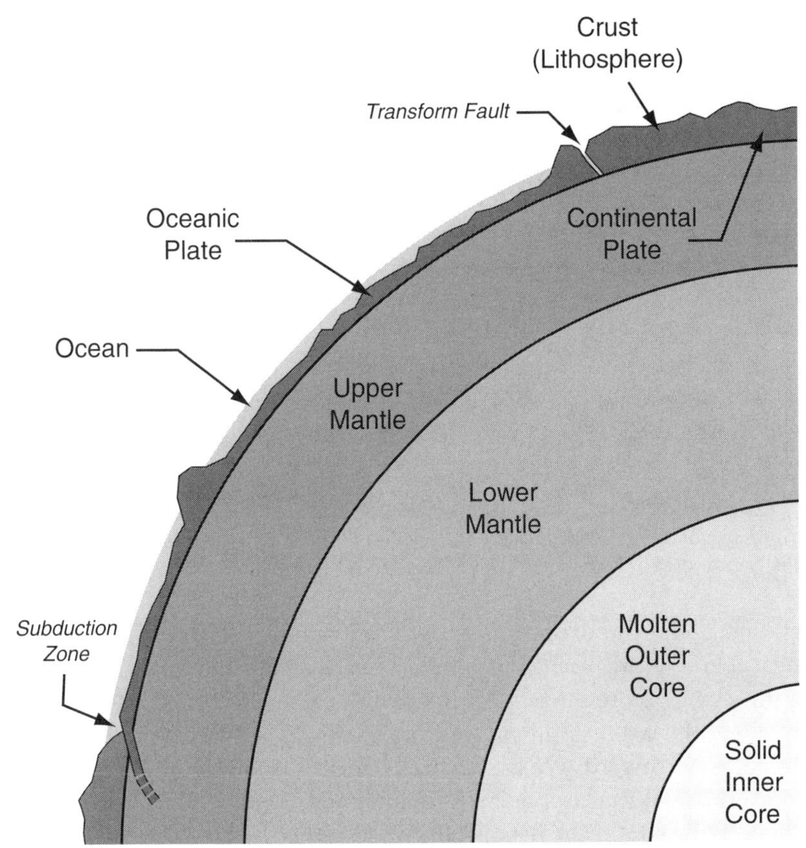

Cross section of the earth. A transform fault occurs when two tectonic plates slide horizontally past each other. A subduction zone occurs when one plate slides under another. The San Andreas Fault is a transform fault.

Jose, causing the famous Loma Prieta earthquake that collapsed freeways and broke a section of the San Francisco Bay Bridge.

Earthquake faults are a result of a geologic process called plate tectonics. Geologists explain that the earth's crust is broken into a number of rigid crustal plates that ride on top of a viscous layer inside the earth known as the mantle. The San Andreas Fault lies at the interface between two of these massive crustal plates: the Pacific Plate to the west and the North American Plate to the east. As these two plates collide, pressure builds at the interface until, in a sudden release of energy we call an earthquake, the two plates slip past each other to relieve the stress.

Because the motion of the plates along the San Andreas Fault is primarily sideways, it is known as a transform fault. Where one plate is

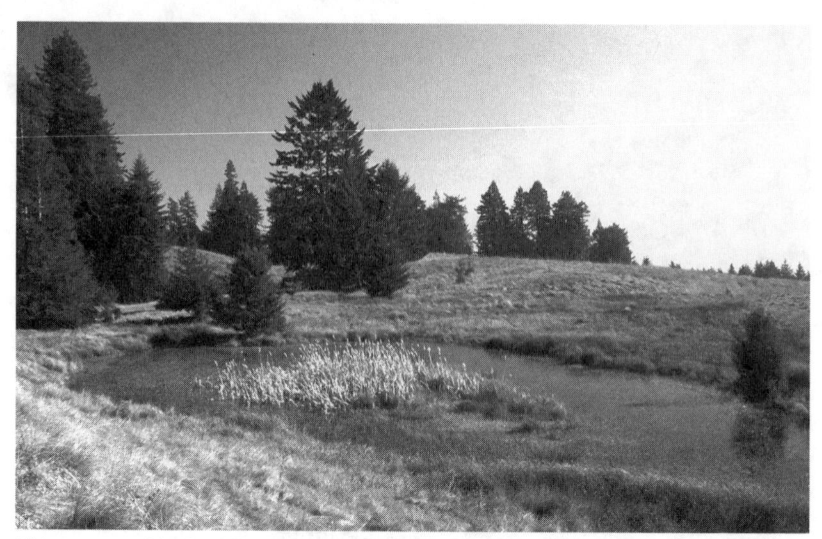

This sag pond in the hills above Fort Ross was formed when the ground sank along the San Andreas Fault.

sliding under the other, it is known as a subduction zone. Shell Beach near Jenner is an excellent example of an ancient subduction zone from a time long before the San Andreas Fault came into being.

Over the last 30 million years, the Pacific Plate has moved hundreds of miles northward. We know this because rocks west of the fault near San Francisco match similar formations on the east side that are 300 miles to the south. On average, the relative motion between the plates is about 2 to 4 inches per year. Sometimes, though, the movement is much greater. During the 1906 earthquake, a section of the fault in Point Reyes moved as much as 21 feet in just a few minutes!

The rugged profile of the Sonoma Coast is the result of constant erosion by water and wind. The erosive power of waves washes away softer rock from seaside cliffs, leaving behind isolated formations of more resistant rock, called sea stacks, surrounded by water. Unstable cliffs regularly crumble into the sea, littering the surf with half-submerged rocky outcroppings. Sonoma cliffs are notoriously dangerous. Despite numerous posted warning signs, people are killed or injured every year in falls from cliff edges.

As the Pacific Plate moves northward, it is pushing the coastline upwards. At various points along the coast, sea stacks that once lay in the ocean now rest on dry land hundreds of feet higher. Two excellent examples are visible on Sonoma Coast State Beach just north of Shell Beach.

Early History of the Coast

Over the years, more nations have laid claims to Sonoma County than anywhere else in the United States. Before the Stars and Stripes, the flags of England, Russia, Spain, the Mexican Empire, the Republic of Mexico, and the California Republic all flew over this coast.

The first inhabitants, though, didn't carry a flag. For at least 7,000 years this land was the domain of Native Americans. At the time of European contact, it was split between two major Indian cultures. The Coast Miwok lived from about Shell Beach south to the Golden Gate, while the Pomo lived north on into Mendocino County.

Although they sometimes bartered with each other, the two cultures evolved separately and spoke vastly different languages. Unlike their brethren on the Great Plains, neither the Miwok nor the Pomo were nomadic tribesmen. Amid such fertile surroundings there was little need to migrate in search of food. They lived instead in small tribelets with well-defined boundaries. They were renown for their exquisite basketmaking skills. The Pomo in particular carried the art of basketry to its highest levels in America.

Juan Rodríguez Cabrillo, a Portuguese explorer under the command of the viceroy of New Spain, was the first European to intrude on this idyllic setting. In 1542 his expedition, searching for the mythical Northwest Passage, sighted land near the future site of Fort Ross. Though he was undoubtedly the first European to view the Sonoma Coast, Cabrillo died during the voyage and reports of his expedition were soon forgotten.

The first European to set foot on Sonoma County soil may well have been the English buccaneer Francis Drake. In the summer of 1579, after a year of plundering Spanish ships in the Pacific, he landed on the California coast to repair his leaking ship, *Golden Hind*. For five weeks, Drake and his men explored the land. They befriended the local Indians, and when he left, Drake posted "a plate of brasse, fast nailed to a great and firme post," claiming the land for the Queen.

Unfortunately, Drake's logbook is lost in antiquity, so the precise spot of his landing is unknown. Every sandbar from San Diego to Eureka has at one time or another claimed him as its own. Two of the most likely spots are Bodega Bay and Drake's Bay. (A minority opinion in favor of San Francisco Bay seems based on little more than wishful thinking.) Though many scholars favor Drake's Bay, Bodega Bay more closely matches the historical record. It is also the better harbor, a fact not likely to be lost on an experienced seaman like Drake.

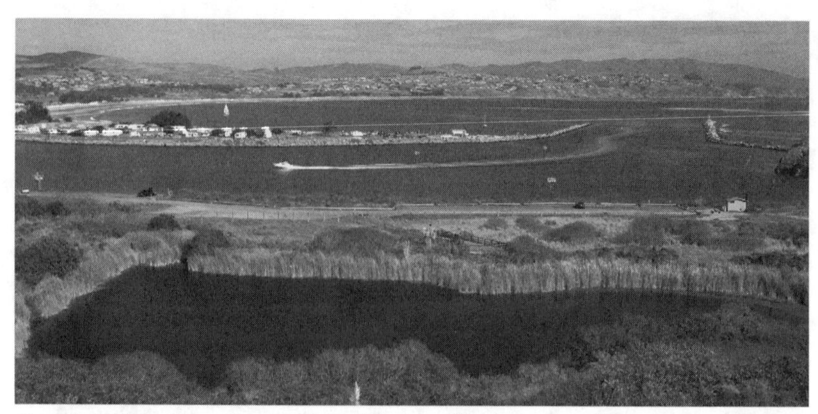

Campbell Cove along the east side of Bodega Head may have been the site of Francis Drake's landing in 1579. The 12-story deep pond in the foreground is Hole-in-the-Head, the lone remnant of an ill-conceived 1960s nuclear power plant.

After Drake, Europeans virtually ignored California for 200 years. In 1775, the Spanish explorer Juan Francisco de la Bodega y Quadra landed briefly at Bodega Bay and thereby conferred its name. Not until Russian settlement in the early 1800s, however, did the Sonoma Coast become of serious interest to Europeans. The Russians desperately needed a steady supply of fruits and vegetables for their Alaskan seal-hunting colonies. Aleksandr Baranov, manager of these colonies, sent expeditions south to hunt sea otters and scout sites for an agricultural colony along the coast north of San Francisco. Ivan Kuskov built a temporary site at Bodega Bay in 1809 and returned in 1812 to found a permanent settlement at Fort Ross. Though the Spanish at San Francisco protested loudly, they were never strong enough to attempt a forcible eviction. In fact, San Francisco was such a remote outpost that the locals tended to ignore the protestations emanating from colonial headquarters in faraway Mexico. Surreptitious trading was common, and in later years, Spanish officials were even occasionally invited to celebrations at the fort.

The Russians occupied Fort Ross for nearly 30 years, never firing a shot in anger. It never lived up to its agricultural promise, but the harvest of sea otter furs was initially profitable. By the 1830s, though, the otters had been nearly exterminated. Debts mounted year by year until the Russians finally withdrew. They sold the fort to John Sutter and abandoned California in 1841.

Mexico had been alarmed at the Russian incursion. To prevent further foreign expansion they vowed to settle the north coast as quickly as possible. Throughout the 1830s and early 1840s, the government made numerous land grants to encourage settlement. In 1840 Stephen Smith received the 35,000-acre Bodega Rancho, stretching from the Russian River south to Estero Americano. The 61-year-old Yankee sea captain settled the land with his 16-year-old Peruvian bride, Manuella. Farther north, German immigrants Charles Meyer and Ernest Rufus in 1846 received the 18,000-acre German Rancho covering the coast from Salt Point to Gualala. Between these two lay the massive Muniz Rancho, awarded to Manuel Torres in 1845.

The rancho period in Sonoma County was destined to be brief. The era of American westward migration had begun, and the newcomers resented a system that locked them out of land ownership. The Bear Flag Revolt of 1846 began in the nearby town of Sonoma, and for 25 days in June and July of that year, California existed as an independent republic. Even after the United States annexed the territory and proclaimed the land grants to be valid, the newcomers ignored them. Most grants were eventually sold off piecemeal by owners unwilling to endure years of protracted legal battles and occasional gunplay with squatters on their lands.

Starting in the 1860s and lasting until a narrow-gauge railroad was put through to the Russian River in the late 1880s, the Sonoma Coast was a shipping center for timber from the nearby redwood forests. There were no real ports along this coast. Instead, lumber was loaded onto schooners from such tiny outports as Duncan's Landing, Fort Ross Cove, Timber Cove, and Stewart's Point. Captains of large vessels scornfully called them "doghole ports" because they were allegedly barely large enough for a dog to turn around. The small, two-masted lumber schooners were invariably piloted by seasoned Scandinavian captains used to maneuvering in the cramped confines of Norwegian fjords.

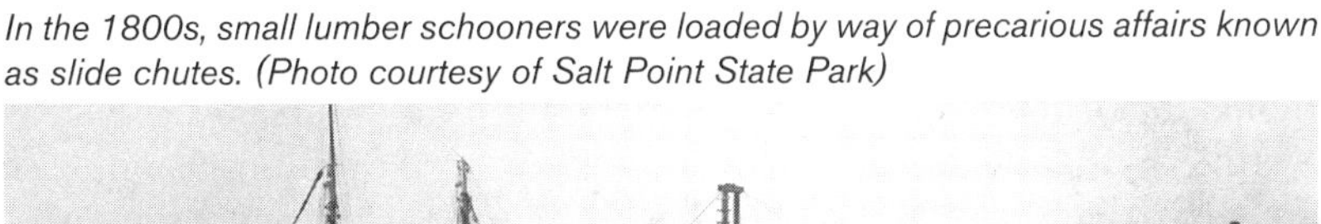

In the 1800s, small lumber schooners were loaded by way of precarious affairs known as slide chutes. (Photo courtesy of Salt Point State Park)

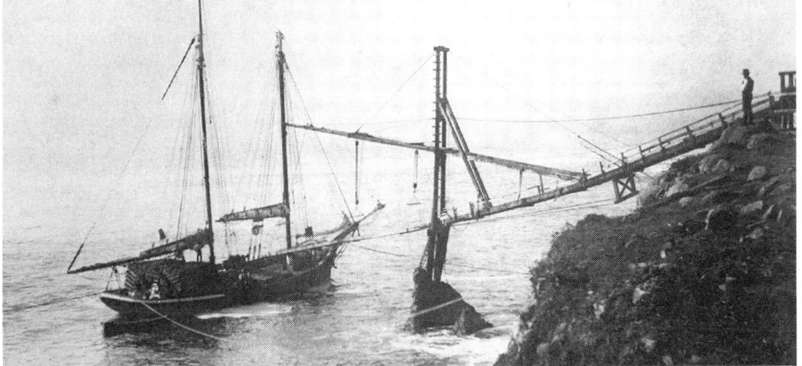

A Graveyard of Ships

Over the years, the rugged shores of Sonoma County have contributed to more than their share of ship disasters. Frequent fogs, rough seas, and a rocky coastline create treacherous conditions for unwary seamen. The latter half of the 19th century was a particularly deadly time. In those days before automobiles and paved highways, ocean travel was the routine method of transportation for both passengers and cargoes along the coast. With only the most rudimentary navigational equipment, courageous captains regularly put their small schooners into doghole ports under extremely difficult conditions.

The annals are full of stories of Sonoma County shipwrecks. In many cases only terse accounts remain, revealing little of the terrors for those unlucky souls involved: "*Ellen H. Wood*, brig, wrecked at Salt Point, 1859, 4 dead; *Hannah Louise*, schooner, capsized at Russian Gulch, 1872, 1 dead; *Liberty*, schooner, wrecked at Timber Cove, 1872, 1 dead; *Mary D. Pomeroy*, schooner, capsized in a gale and washed ashore at Salt Point, 1879, 15 missing; *Two Brothers*, schooner, capsized at Bodega Head, 1883, 4 dead; *Volunteer*, 4-masted schooner, wrecked at Bodega Head, 1906, 3 dead, including captain's two children, when his wife ordered their lifeboat into the dangerous surf instead of open sea."

Sometimes, the stories have happier endings. In 1908 the passenger steamship *Pomona* struck a submerged reef and foundered at Fort Ross. The Call family, owners of the ranch at Fort Ross, came down the bluff to help save the 84 passengers and crew.

Time has erased all evidence of most of these wrecks, but an occasional trace still remains. The 386-foot steamship freighter *Norlina*, built in 1909, ran aground at Gerstle Cove in heavy fog the night of August 4, 1926. Her rusted hulk still rests in shallow water south of the cove, visible at low tide to those who know where to look.

Schooners anchored in these outports were loaded by way of a precarious affair known as a slide chute—a wooden ramp supported by pillars that extended down from a high bluff to the ship's deck. Boards were individually launched down the ramp to the waiting hands of a crewman on deck. A series of brakes was supposed to slow the boards, but mishaps were common, especially in rough weather. The slide chute was used to load everything from lumber to supplies to the occasional intrepid passenger. If a storm came up, the schooner would have to put to sea quickly to avoid being dashed on the rocks.

In 1873, George W. Call purchased 15,000 acres around Fort Ross and established the Call Ranch. The site of the former Russian outpost was sold to the California Historical Landmarks Committee in 1903 and turned over to the State in 1906. Sonoma Coast State Park was acquired in 1934 and Salt Point State Park in 1968.

Exploring the Coast

The main road linking the various communities along the Sonoma Coast is a winding, two-lane adventure called State Highway 1. Don't expect to get anywhere along it in a hurry. The combination of twisting hillside curves, drivers dazzled by the scenery, and the occasional bicyclist, pedestrian, or loose farm animal make it unsafe to hurry. Take it easy, plan a leisurely journey, and enjoy the drive. The road includes numerous turnouts that allow you to safely observe the spectacular views and let more impatient traffic pass.

There are two popular routes west to the coast from US Highway 101. The southern route departs the freeway in Santa Rosa at the Highway 12 exit, heads west to Sebastopol, and continues along the Bodega Highway to Highway 1 just south of Bodega Bay. The northern route exits at River Road, heads west to Guerneville, then continues along Highway 116 to Highway 1 at Jenner. Both routes are especially scenic, and both can be heavily traveled, particularly on summer weekends.

Though it is possible to see the entire coast in a single day, a better choice is to plan at least two or three days. Numerous accommodations can be found all along the coast at places such as Bodega Bay, Jenner, Timber Cove, and The Sea Ranch. For the more adventurous, campgrounds suitable for tent or RV camping are located at Sonoma Coast, Fort Ross, and Salt Point State Parks, as well as in Doran and Gualala Point Regional Parks and several private campgrounds. You may also choose to combine your visit with a tour of the exceptional

The Tides Restaurant in Bodega Bay was prominently featured in Alfred Hitchcock's 1963 thriller, The Birds. *After having been remodeled twice in the intervening years, it remains a favorite spot for hungry travelers.*

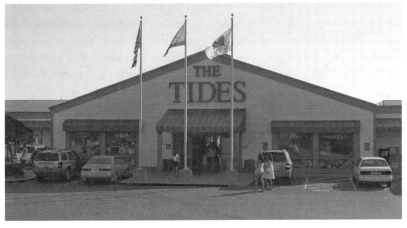

Sonoma County wine country. For touring recommendations, stop at the Santa Rosa Convention and Visitors Bureau in Railroad Square at 9 Fourth Street, Santa Rosa, 800-404-7673, or visit their web site at www.visitsantarosa.com.

A typical coastal tour starts from Bodega Highway out of Sebastopol. The route winds through apple orchards and pasturelands to the town of Bodega (not to be confused with Bodega Bay), half a mile east of the Highway 1 junction. Captain Stephen Smith built California's first steam-powered sawmill here in the 1840s. The town is home to art galleries and antique shops along with several historic buildings. The most prominent is St. Teresa's Church, built in 1859 and the subject of a famous Ansel Adams photograph. Behind the church is Potter School House, featured in Alfred Hitchcock's classic 1963 thriller, *The Birds*. A historic cemetery west of town is the final resting place for many early area residents.

This region was originally settled by Russian pioneers in the early 1800s. They built the farming community of Kuskov along the present Salmon Creek Road to help supply their settlement at Fort Ross. No trace of Kuskov or its inhabitants remains today.

After leaving Bodega, turn right at the Highway 1 junction. The road winds 4 miles through Cheney Creek Canyon to Bodega Bay, centerpiece of the southern coast. Here you will find shops, markets, restaurants, and accommodations. Spud Point Marina on Westshore Road is home to a large fishing fleet. From December through April, wildlife enthusiasts converge on Bodega Head as a premier spot for whale watching. The University of California also operates a marine laboratory and refuge here. The entire Bodega Bay area is an important stopover for migratory birds and draws hordes of birders during migration.

Doran Beach, at the southern end of the harbor, is the site of a county park and campground. The headquarters for Sonoma Coast State Park are located at Salmon Creek Beach, just north of town. This long, sandy beach is a popular destination on hot summer weekends. For part of the winter, the cypress and eucalyptus groves adjacent to nearby Bodega Dunes are home to thousands of monarch butterflies.

State beaches lie interspersed with private property all along the coast to Jenner. Portuguese Beach and Duncan's Cove are popular rock fishing and surf netting spots. Shell Beach is a frequent destination for school field trips to explore tidepool marine life. And for much of the year, a large seal colony is a fixture along the Russian River at the north end of Goat Rock Beach.

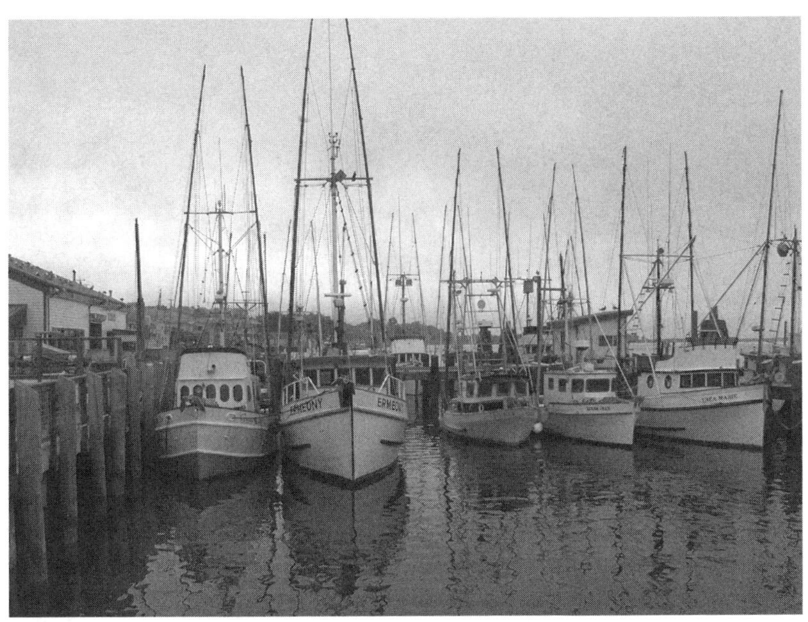

The town of Bodega Bay is home to the largest fishing fleet between San Francisco and Eureka.

The town of Jenner sits above the mouth of the Russian River. Originally a lumber town, it is now home to a community of artists and fishermen. Until the highway bridge was built in the 1930s, the only way across the river here was by ferry.

North of Jenner the highway quickly winds 600 feet above the sea. Known as Sonoma's Lost Coast, this shoreline is accessible only to the dedicated hiker. Come properly equipped and pay attention to tide tables if you want to explore this beautiful but isolated region.

Eleven miles north of Jenner lies Fort Ross, site of the first permanent settlement along the California coast north of San Francisco. The restored fort now stands as part of Fort Ross State Historic Park. There are also several miles of hiking trails within the park.

Just beyond Fort Ross is the town of Timber Cove, founded as a lumber community in the late 1800s. It was once a main shipping point for cordwood, fence posts, tanbark, and railroad ties. A Timber Cove landmark is the famous Bufano peace statue, *The Expanding Universe,* at the Timber Cove Inn. The internationally acclaimed artist and pacifist Benjamin Bufano erected the sculpture in 1965 as a monument to the folly of war.

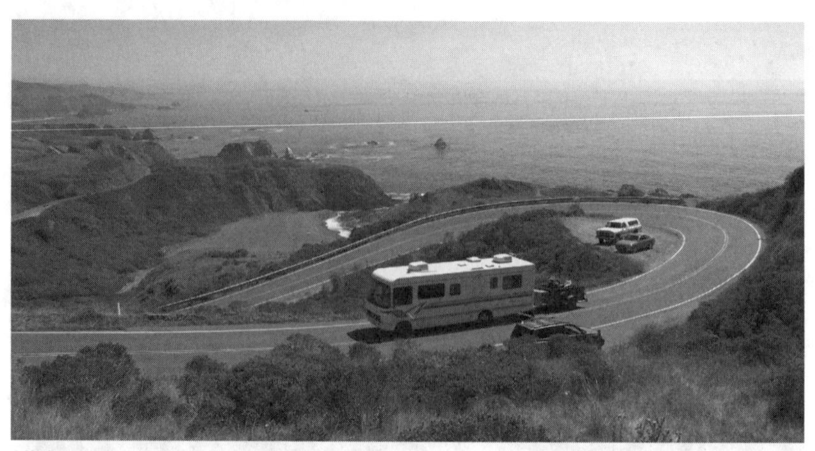

Highway 1 between Jenner and Fort Ross is a winding, two-lane road that climbs as high as 600 feet above the sea.

California State Park System Rules and Regulations

The following rules and regulations apply to all units of the California State Park System. These rules and regulations protect park areas for the enjoyment of future generations as well as for the convenience and safety of the park visitors. To ensure your visit is a pleasant one, please observe the following:

NATURAL SCENERY, PLANTS AND ANIMAL LIFE are the principal attractions of most state parks. They are integral parts of the ecosystem and natural community. As such, they are protected by Federal, State, and Park laws. Disturbance or destruction of these resources is strictly forbidden.

LOADED FIREARMS AND HUNTING are not allowed in units of the State Parks System. Possession of loaded firearms or air rifles is prohibited. Exceptions are for hunting in recreation areas that have been designated by the State Park and Recreation Commission.

DEAD AND DOWN WOOD is part of the natural condition. Decayed vegetation forms humus and assists the growth of trees and other plants. For this reason the gathering of down wood is prohibited. Fuel is sold in the parks for your convenience. (When considered a hazard, down wood is removed by park personnel.)

FIRES are permitted only in facilities provided for this purpose. This is necessary to prevent disastrous fires. Portable stoves may be used in designated areas. It is the responsibility of every visitor to use extreme caution with any burning materials, including tobacco. All fireworks are prohibited.

ANIMALS, including cats, cannot be turned loose in park units. All animals, other than grazing animals, must be under immediate physical control. Dogs must be on

Six-thousand-acre Salt Point State Park lies north of Timber Cove. Its varied terrain includes forested mountains, a sandy ocean cove, and sculptured rocky promontories. Salt Point is a popular site for abalone diving, as well as camping, hiking, picnicking, and horseback riding. Directly adjacent is Kruse Rhododendron State Reserve, donated to the State by Edward P. E. Kruse in 1933. The trails through this park are especially picturesque when the rhododendrons bloom in May.

Near the northern end of the county lies a planned community, The Sea Ranch. The town was founded in the mid-1960s and includes a golf course, lodge, and over a thousand upscale homes that have been designed to blend with the coastal landscape.

a tended leash no more than 6 feet or confined in an enclosed vehicle, tent, or pen. Unless posted to the contrary, dogs, other than those that assist the permanently disabled, are prohibited on trails, beaches, and wherever posted. Visitors with vicious, dangerous, noisy, or disturbing animals will be ejected from park units.

NOISE—Engine driven electric generators that can disturb others, may be operated only between the hours 10 A.M. and 8 P.M. Loud disturbing noise is prohibited at all times, as is disturbing those asleep between 10 P.M. and 6 A.M.

ALL VEHICLE TRAVEL must be confined to designated roads or areas. The speed for all vehicles is 15 miles per hour in camp, picnic, utility, or headquarters areas and areas of general assemblage. Parking is permitted only in designated areas. Blocking parking spaces is prohibited.

CAMPSITE USE must be paid for in advance. To hold a campsite, it must be reserved or occupied. To prevent encroachment on others the District Superintendent may regulate the limits of each campsite. Checkout time is 12:00 noon. In order to provide for the greatest number of visitors possible. The camping limit in any one campground is 30 days per calendar year.

REFUSE, including garbage, cigarettes, paper boxes, bottles, ashes and other rubbish, shall be placed only in designated receptacles. Your pleasure and pride in your parks will be enhanced when they are kept clean.

PLEASE clean up after yourself so that others may enjoy the beauty of these parks.

Climate

Mark Twain (probably apocryphally) said "the coldest winter I ever spent was one summer in San Francisco." The English buccaneer Francis Drake described the area as a land of "stynking fogges," and complained that despite landing in the height of summer, "were wee continually visited with like nipping colds." Clearly, the warm, sunny beaches of Southern California are absent here, but despite the bad publicity, the Sonoma Coast is not as harsh as it might sound. The rainy season is mainly confined between the months of October and March. Winter temperatures rarely approach freezing, though with the frequent winds it often seems colder. Summers can actually be quite pleasant when the fog recedes. At these times, a trip to the coast can be a welcome respite from the 100$^+$-degree temperatures inland.

Regardless of the time of year, come prepared for cool, windy weather. Bring a sweater or jacket and leave it in the car if you don't need it. In winter, additional apparel should include a hat, gloves, and water-repellent rain shell. Don't be fooled by warmer weather inland. Even a few miles from the coast the temperature can be 20°F higher. At times, the town of Bodega Bay can be bathed in warm sunlight while across the sand dunes, Salmon Creek Beach and the northern coast can be fogged in. It is also wise to bring sunscreen or similar protection. Fog or clouds offer little shelter from harmful rays, so use sunscreen even on an overcast day.

The cold waters of the Sonoma Coast are not suitable for casual swimming. Strong waves and rip currents can make it dangerous even to play in the surf. Diehard surfers and divers should venture into the ocean only if they are in good physical condition, adequately trained, and properly equipped with wet suits. Never enter the water alone!

Animal Life

Land Mammals. Early travelers were quick to note the variety of wildlife inhabiting the Sonoma Coast. Kyrill Khlebnikov, a Russian who visited Fort Ross in the early 1800s, observed "bears, lynx, ordinary wolves, and the small ones which the Spaniards call coyotes." The most majestic and dangerous animal was the California grizzly bear. Hunted mercilessly, it was driven to extinction by the end of the 19th century. It somewhat ironically remains a fixture on the State flag, first flown over the nearby Sonoma barracks during the Bear Flag Revolt of 1846.

Mammals commonly found here today include black-tailed deer, raccoons, striped skunks, squirrels, chipmunks, rabbits, field mice, and a host of other rodents. More reclusive are the bobcat, gray fox, badger, and the rare black bear and mountain lion. Raccoons, skunks, foxes, and deer can be persistent pests in certain coastal campgrounds, so store food in secure containers when not in use.

Birds. For at least part of the year the Sonoma Coast is home to hundreds of species of birds. The more common residents include gulls, cormorants, herons, egrets, pelicans, ospreys, doves, quail, ravens, vultures, hawks, and a wide variety of waterfowl and songbirds. Populations are highest during the fall and spring migrations. Bodega Bay, an important stop along the migration path, is a favorite spot for bird watching.

Marine Mammals. The most visible marine mammals are the numerous harbor seals that reside along the coast, especially at the mouth of the Russian River. Although they may appear docile, seals frighten easily and can inflict serious bites. They are protected by the Marine Mammal Protection Act, which makes it unlawful to feed, harass, or

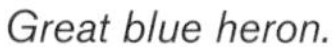
Great blue heron.

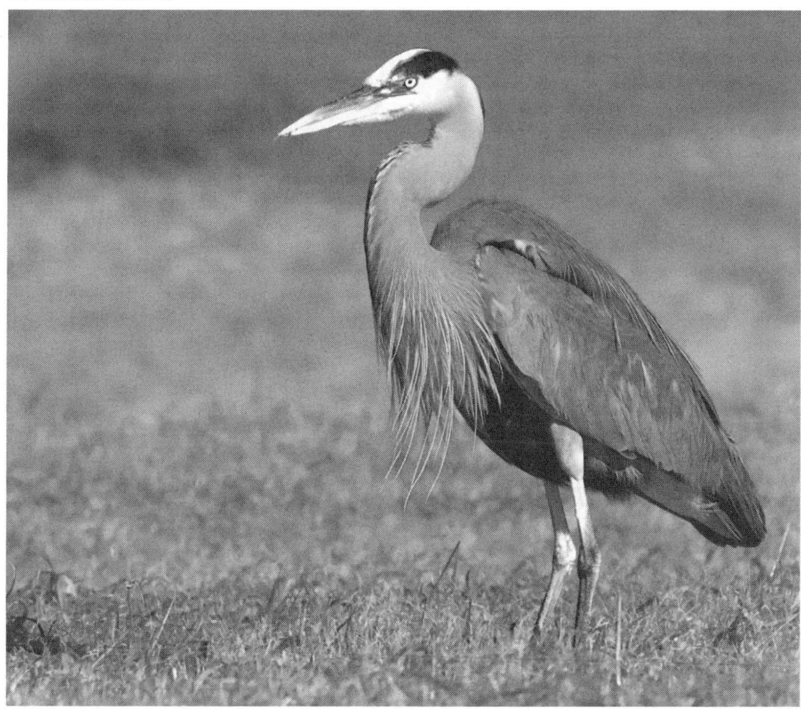

approach them too closely. Whales, dolphins, porpoises, and sea lions are also protected by this act. On summer weekends, volunteers from the Stewards of the Coast and Redwoods are normally on hand at Goat Rock Beach to answer questions, loan binoculars, and keep the unwary visitor from approaching the seals too closely.

Bodega Head is an ideal spot to watch the semi-annual migration of the Pacific gray whale. The southward journey occurs in December and January. At the front of the pack are the pregnant females, racing to reach the warm waters of Baja California in time for the birth of their young. They are followed by mature males, non-pregnant females, and finally the juveniles. Calves are born the first two weeks in January. The northward migration takes place at a more leisurely pace starting as temperatures rise in February. First to leave are the females who became pregnant on the southern journey, followed by the males. Last

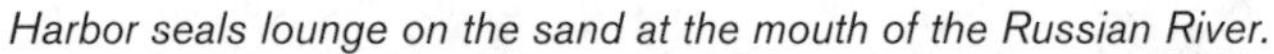
Harbor seals lounge on the sand at the mouth of the Russian River.

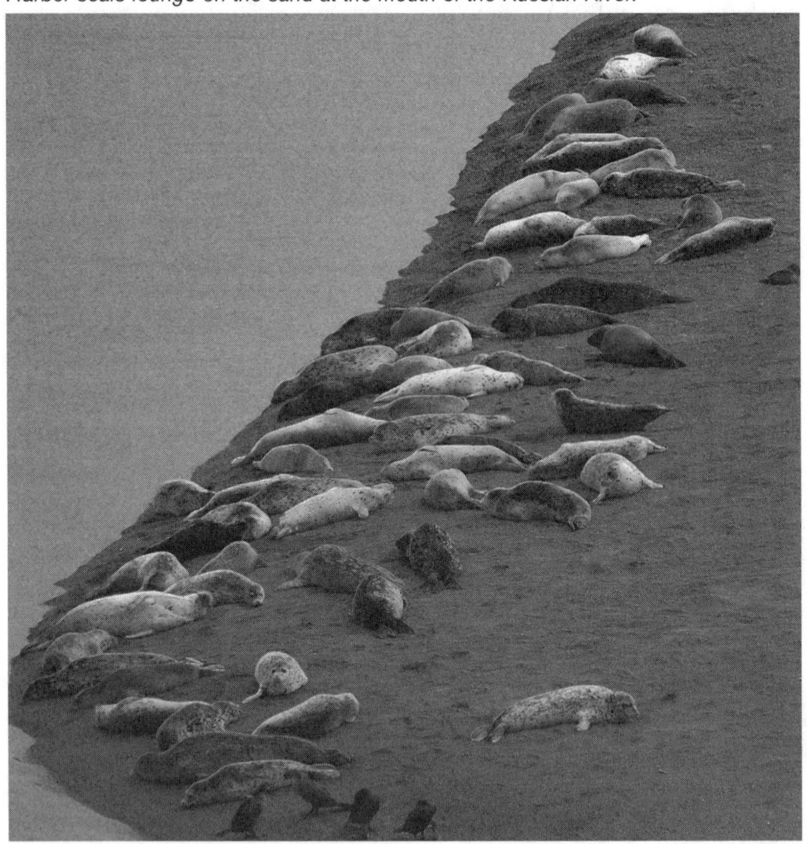

to leave, during the month of April, are the new mothers and calves. It is believed that the whales do not feed during the entire migration period and can lose a third of their body weight by the time they return to their Arctic feeding grounds.

Fish and Shellfish. A wide variety of sea life abounds along the coast. In rocky areas, common fish and mollusks include rock cod, ling cod, cabezon, sculpin, abalone, and mussels. Those off sandy beaches include perch, smelt, halibut, sanddabs, and flounder. Clams found in the mud flats of Bodega Harbor include horsenecks, cockles, littlenecks, and Washington. Rock crab and Dungeness crab can also be caught in the Bodega Harbor and jetty area.

Anyone 16 years of age or older who takes any kind of fish, mollusk, amphibian, or crustacean must possess a valid California fishing license. Refer to Fish and Game Regulations for specific information regarding minimum size and limits on specific species. Also, some shellfish, especially mussels, may be poisonous when feeding on the toxic algae that create "red tides" at certain times of the year. Always inquire about quarantines before collecting any shellfish.

Northern California waters are also home to a variety of sharks. The waters around Bodega Bay are at the edge of an important breeding ground for great whites. Seals are a favorite food, and several local attacks have occurred by great whites mistaking a surfer or scuba diver for a seal.

Intertidal Life. The rocky Sonoma shores are host to an abundance of tidal life. Different sets of organisms live in each of the three major intertidal zones. Those with least tolerance to atmospheric exposure live in the low tide zone. More tolerant species live in the mid tide zone, where they may be exposed to air for several hours per day. The most tolerant species live in the high tide zone where they are protected from heavy wave action. Plants and animals of the low tide zone include abalones, sponges, ribbed kelp, anemones, urchins, thatched barnacles, and coralline algae. Those of the mid tide zone include sea palms, mussels, goose barnacles, sea stars, hermit crabs, sea sacks, and aggregated anemones. Periwinkles, limpets, sea lettuce, acorn barnacles, lined shore crabs, and turban snails are typical of life in the high tide zone.

The greatest danger to the intertidal ecology is not the harsh natural environment, but rather the actions of man. Plants and animals exposed to air by the simple act of turning over a rock or moving it higher up the shore will quickly die. Remember these guidelines when exploring tidepool life:

- When looking under rocks, return them to their exact original positions. Animals such as sponges and anemones attached to the underside of rocks will die if left exposed to sun, air, and predators.
- Use a pail or jar to observe free-swimming life, and return it to where you found it when finished.
- Don't try to permanently remove the animals you find. They will quickly die. Remember also that within state parks it is illegal to collect tidepool life.
- The best times for exploring are during low tides. The lowest tides, called spring tides, occur every two weeks near the times of the full moon and new moon. Consult a newspaper or check

Ocean Safety

The rugged Sonoma coast is known for its beauty, but it can also be dangerous. From 1951 through 1990 there were 88 deaths on the coast, most attributed to drowning. The three most common causes are playing in the surf, fishing, and beachcombing. Scrambling along unstable cliffs and abalone diving in rough weather have also contributed their share of deaths.

A phenomenon called "shore break" is particularly treacherous at beaches such as Goat Rock and Wright's Beach. A deep trench just offshore causes a very shallow wave break. The backwash also goes only as far as the wave break. So a person swept into the sea is pulled out only a short distance before being rushed toward shore, then pulled again back to sea. This "washing machine" effect keeps the victim just out of reach of rescuers on shore. As he is swept parallel to shore, he is eventually dashed onto nearby rocks.

Another danger, especially in fall and winter, is "sleeper waves" generated by storms far out to sea. Multiple sets of waves can overlap as they rush to shore. When the peak of one wave coincides with the trough of another, the sea may look calm and visitors may be lulled into a false sense of security. Then a set of waves that are "in phase" may roll in, building to a single wave far larger than most. The rush of water from this enormous wave can quickly sweep victims into the surf where rip currents (currents that flow straight out to sea) pull them far into the ocean.

To avoid becoming the next statistic, remember these simple rules:

- Pay attention to the ocean. Never turn your back to it.
- Avoid the beach area between the surf and the high water mark. Never venture into the surf.
- Always have an avenue of escape. When scrambling along rocks, be aware of the tide and return to safety well before you are cut off from the shore.

the NOAA website at http://tidesandcurrents.noaa.gov/ for the times of low tides on a particular day. Tide tables for the entire year can be purchased at numerous shops along the coast.

- Dress appropriately. Northern California waters are cold, and the algae-covered rocks are extremely slippery. If you intend to venture any distance from shore, wear waterproof rubber-soled boots or shoes. Pick your way carefully among the rocks and be sure of your footing before taking a step. Consider using a hiking staff to help maintain your balance.
- Observe the rules of ocean safety. Stay aware of your surroundings and never turn your back to the sea. Don't let young children explore on their own. Keep track of the incoming tide and return to shore well before your route is cut off by the sea.

- If you are caught in a rip current, don't try to swim back against it. Instead, swim parallel to shore until you are out of the current, then swim back to shore.
- Remember that not all dangers come from the sea. Many people are killed or injured in falls from cliffs. Follow established trails to the water and stay back from cliff edges.

Divers should remember these additional precautions:

- Before leaving for the coast, check the website describing current ocean conditions for Salt Point State Park at www.saltpointoceanconditions.com.
- Upon arrival, check with local park staff or businesses to determine a safe diving location.
- Watch the prospective dive area for at least 20 minutes prior to entering the water to identify water conditions, rip currents, and easy access points. Plan for alternate exits if the sea becomes rough.
- Always take a float (inner tube, dive mat, dive board, or boat) when you dive.
- Never dive alone.
- Let someone know where you will be diving and when you expect to return.
- Diving is strenuous sport. Be in good physical condition and be sure your gear is in good condition.
- Never enter the water if it is too rough. Your life may depend on it.

Hazardous Plants and Animals

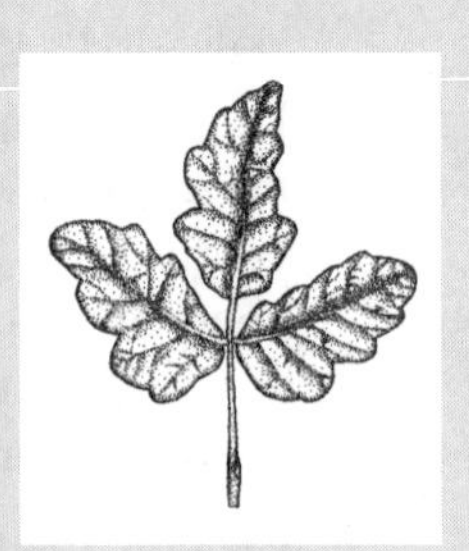

Poison Oak. The one plant you absolutely need to know how to identify is poison oak. Unfortunately it doesn't always look the same. In direct sun, it grows as a shrub, while in shady areas, it grows as a clinging vine. The one commonality is the leaves–they grow in clusters of three leaflets attached to a single stalk. Poison oak is one of the first plants to turn color in the year, becoming brilliant orange or red by late summer. The leaves are gone by winter but the stems are still poisonous, making this a more hazardous time of year.

The toxin in poison oak is an oily substance called urushiol. You don't have to actually touch the plant to get poisoned. If it gets on your clothing or on your dog, you can pick it up through secondary transmission. The oil remains potent on clothing for months or years, so wash contaminated clothing as soon as possible and don't mix other items in the same wash. Also, don't burn poison oak. The urushiol is carried in the smoke, and if inhaled, can cause serious lung poisoning requiring hospitalization.

The best way to deal with poison oak is to avoid it. Stay on trails and learn how to recognize it in the field. Wear long pants and a long-sleeved shirt. If you do get exposed, take a shower as soon as possible, using plenty of soap and lukewarm water. (Don't take a bath, as the oil will just float on top of the bathwater and spread all over your body.)

If you do develop the rash, you can try reducing the itching with cool compresses or a topical application of hydrocortisone. In extreme cases, see your doctor. Treatment with Prednisone, an oral steroid, is usually very effective but can sometimes cause significant side effects.

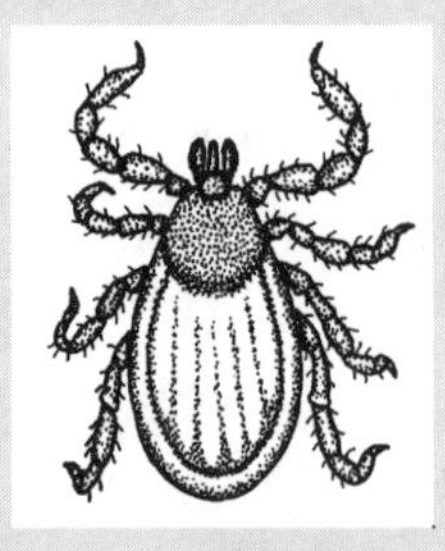

Ticks. Spend any time in the outdoors and you'll eventually encounter a tick. If you know what to do, though, it doesn't have to be an unpleasant experience. Ticks are a leading carrier of diseases, including Lyme disease, Rocky Mountain spotted fever, babesiosis, tularemia, and ehrlichiosis. There are numerous species of ticks, but only a few attach onto humans. The western black-legged tick, Ixodus pacificus, (also known as the deer tick) is the only tick that transmits Lyme disease.

Although tick-borne diseases aren't as prevalent in California as in the Northeast, it's still important to take steps to protect yourself. First, you need to understand that ticks don't fly or jump, although they can drop down from above. Generally, though, they live in grassy areas. A tick will climb to the top of a blade of grass and reach out with its front legs, a behavior called "questing." When an animal or human brushes the grass, the tick grabs on. It may wander around on the host for several hours before attaching and drawing blood.

You can do several things to reduce your risk of a tick bite. First, wear long pants and a long sleeved shirt, and tuck your pants legs inside your socks. Wear light colored clothing to make the ticks more visible, and check yourself regularly. Insect repellents that contain DEET are very effective, but be sure to follow the manufacturer's directions when applying.

If you do find that a tick has attached, you need to remove it. Don't just pull it out, as you will probably cause it to regurgitate and increase your risk of infection. Use fine-tipped tweezers or a specially designed tick removal tool to grasp the tick at the attachment point, and lift straight up. Fortunately, medical evidence indicates that a tick must be attached for at least 24 hours before it transmits Lyme disease, so you don't need to be unnecessarily hasty about removing it.

You may not always know that you have been bitten. In the larval and nymph stages, the tick is very small. Even if you haven't noticed a tick on you, if you discover a bulls-eye-shaped rash on your body within a few weeks after being outdoors, seek medical advice. This is a telltale sign of Lyme disease. However, you can take comfort in knowing that according to the Sonoma County Department of Health Services, fewer than 3% of local ticks are infected with Lyme disease.

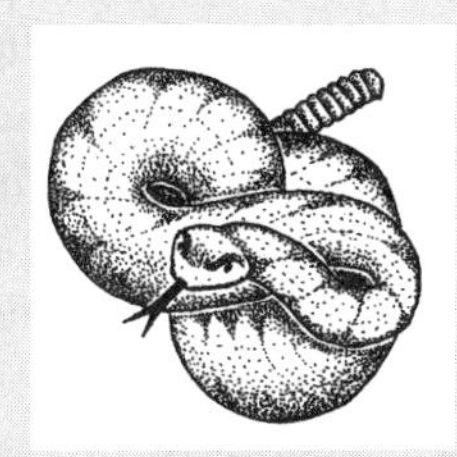

Rattlesnakes. The stereophonic reverberation of a rattlesnake's warning rattle is a sound you won't soon forget. But the reality is that you are unlikely to ever hear it. Rattlesnakes are reclusive creatures that go to great lengths to avoid people. I've been hiking Sonoma County trails for more than 30 years and have only had a few encounters, none serious. That doesn't mean rattlesnakes are not out there, only that they don't want to see you any more than you want to see them.

Snakes prefer dry, rocky, or grassy areas. You can also find them under logs or anywhere rodents are likely to live. To minimize your risk when out hiking, wear boots or shoes, not sandals, and stay on trails as much as possible. Step on top of logs and rocks, not over them, and don't reach into dark places you can't see into. If absolutely necessary to do so, first use a hiking staff to poke around and make sure there are no snakes or other critters inside. If you do encounter a snake, move away slowly. Most bites occur because the snake was surprised or felt threatened.

If you are bitten, seek immediate medical treatment. A snake won't always inject venom when it bites, but don't take any chances. And remember that not every snake out there is a rattlesnake. You're more likely to encounter a harmless garter snake or king snake than a rattlesnake, so avoid the temptation to club any snake you see.

Using this Book

This book is designed to help you get the most out of your visit to the Sonoma Coast and Russian River. It is organized by park, with a dedicated chapter for each state park plus an additional chapter for the regional parks. Each chapter includes detailed information on the park's history, natural history, points of interest, and hiking trails. I have also included sidebars throughout the book that describe particularly interesting facts and features.

Many readers will want to know about each park's hiking trails—which ones are best for families, which are more challenging, and what to see along the way. I have included detailed descriptions for 25 hikes. I mapped each hike using a GPS receiver, recording waypoint locations for numerous sights along the way. These coordinates, along with each feature's description and suggested waypoint name, are presented in easy-to-use tables following the hike's description. To maximize your hiking experience, enter these coordinates into your own GPS receiver and use them to help you navigate.

Each trail description starts with an overview of the trail, directions to the trailhead, total trail length, estimated hiking time, and level of difficulty. Coming up with trail difficulty ratings and hiking times is always subjective. If you're used to hiking in the Grand Canyon, none of the trails in this book will seem overly difficult. If you're not in great shape, though, some of them may be too difficult to attempt. I myself tend to hike trails at a leisurely pace so I can enjoy the outdoors as well as get some exercise.

For the trails in this book, I have defined difficulty as follows:

Easy: A short, relatively level trail that can be completed by a person in average physical condition in less than an hour. Generally suitable for families with children.

Moderate: A trail typically from 1 to 3 miles in length, with an elevation change less than 500 feet and no excessively steep slopes or sandy sections. The trail could include an occasional stream crossing that requires you to rock-hop across it, or it could include rough, washed out segments. May not be advisable for pre-teen children.

Strenuous: A trail longer than 3 miles with noticeable elevation changes, or a shorter trail with more than 1000 feet elevation change or significant stretches through soft sand. May include steep sections that require extra care in hiking. For these trails, everyone in your party should be an experienced hiker in good physical condition.

Hiking times assume you are in average physical condition and are not out to break records on your hike. For longer hikes I have added a reasonable amount of time for rest breaks, although lunch breaks would be extra. I typically estimate walking speeds of no more than 2 miles per hour, and half that speed over soft sand. Times are also adjusted to account for trails with significant uphill or downhill stretches.

All the trails described in this book have been mapped using Garmin GPS receivers. My current receiver of choice is a GPSMap 60CSx because its sensitive receiver works well even under heavy tree cover. Some trails were mapped with a GPSMap 60Cs or an eTrex Vista. I created the trail maps in this book from the GPS tracklogs using the techniques described in my book, *Outdoor Navigation with GPS*. I measured distances using the GPS odometer, which is generally more accurate than a manual pedometer. All GPS waypoints were recorded in the field using the GPS receiver. Remember, however, that GPS will seldom measure your position to better than 20 feet, and under heavy tree cover you can get errors in excess of 50 feet. So don't expect to punch the coordinates from this book into your GPS receiver and have it guide you any closer than that to your intended destination.

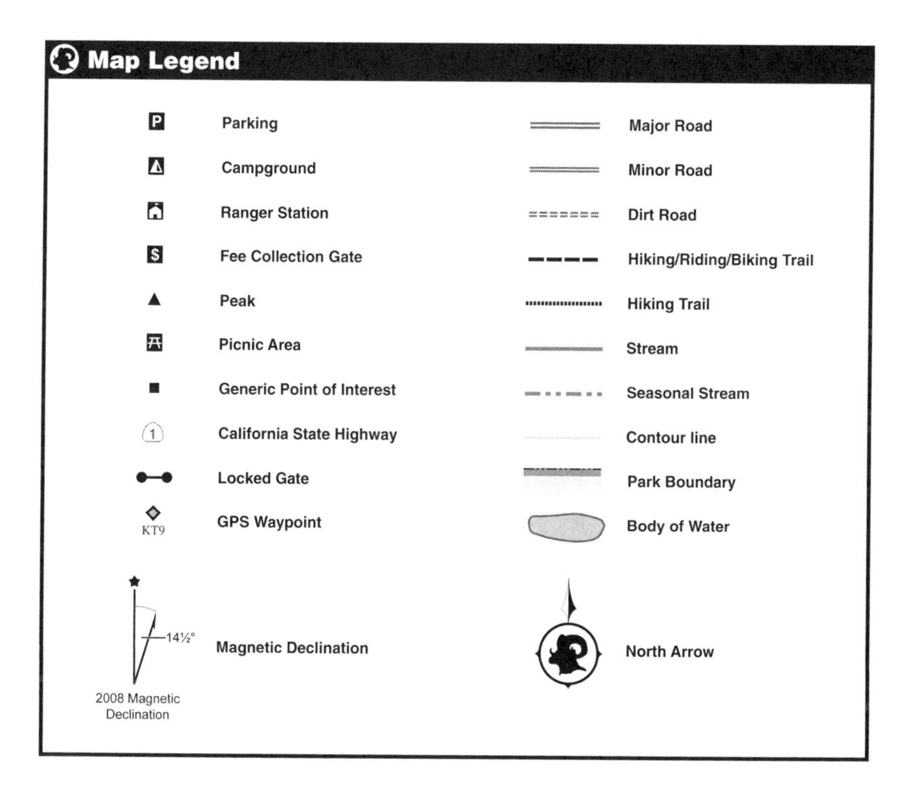

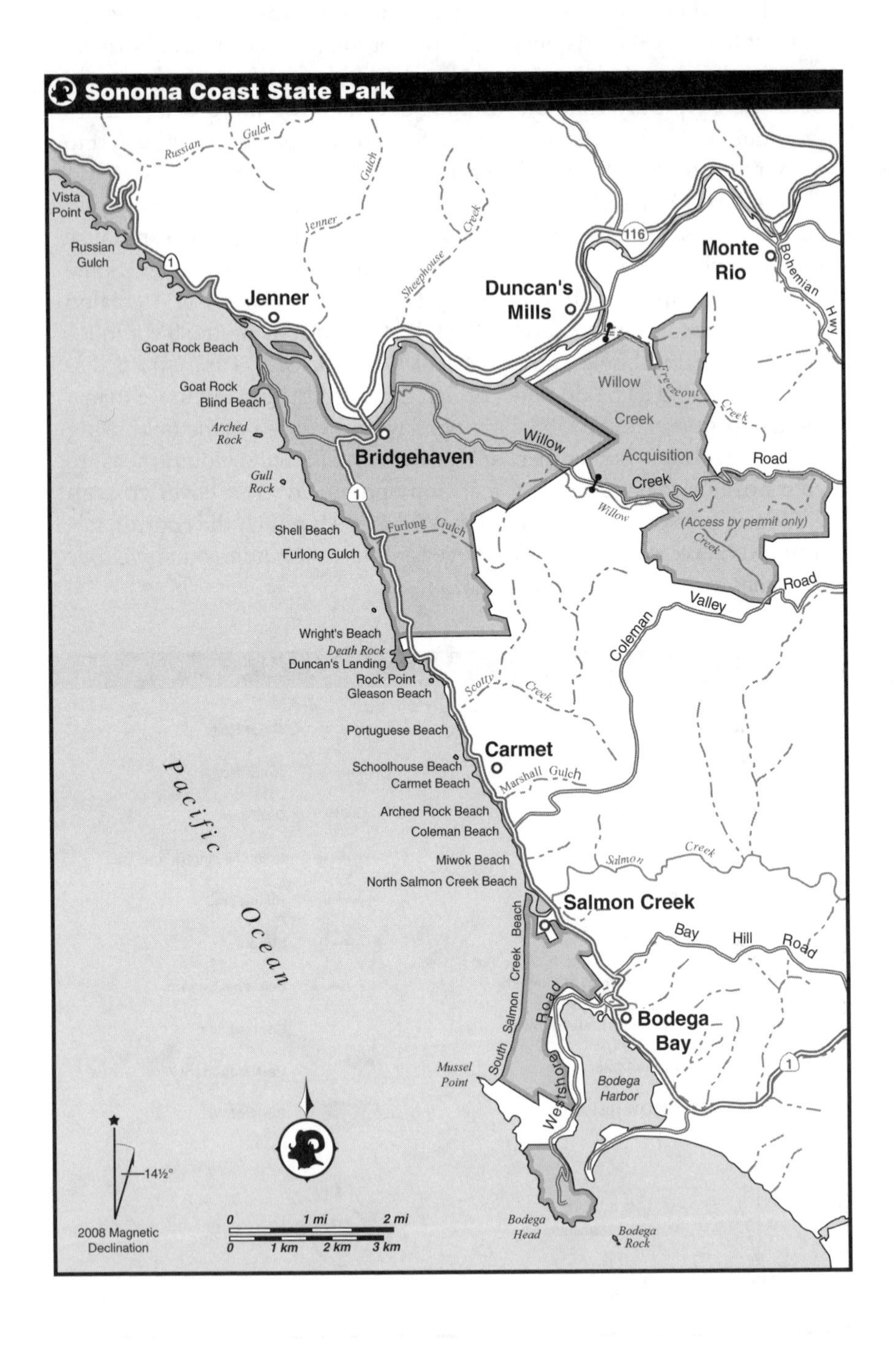

Sonoma Coast State Park
Russian Gulch
Jenner Gulch
Sheephouse Creek
Vista Point
Russian Gulch
1
116
Monte Rio
Bohemian Hwy
Duncan's Mills
Jenner
Goat Rock Beach
Goat Rock
Blind Beach
Arched Rock
Willow Creek Acquisition
Freezeout Creek
Road
Bridgehaven
Willow
Creek
Willow
Gull Rock
(Access by permit only)
Creek
Shell Beach
Furlong Gulch
Furlong Gulch
Road
Valley
Coleman
Wright's Beach
Death Rock
Duncan's Landing
Rock Point
Gleason Beach
Scotty Creek
Portuguese Beach
Carmet
Schoolhouse Beach
Carmet Beach
Marshall Gulch
Arched Rock Beach
Coleman Beach
Miwok Beach
North Salmon Creek Beach
Salmon Creek
Pacific Ocean
Salmon Creek
Bay Hill Road
South Salmon Creek Beach
Road
Westshore
Bodega Bay
Mussel Point
Bodega Harbor
14½°
2008 Magnetic Declination
0 1 mi 2 mi
0 1 km 2 km 3 km
Bodega Head
Bodega Rock

Chapter 2

Sonoma Coast State Park

When you first see the empty shores of Sonoma Coast State Park, you may not believe it is California's second most popular state park. In 2006 it hosted over 3 million visitors, making it busier than such familiar sites as Point Reyes National Seashore and Mount Tamalpais State Park. Even California's crown jewel, Yosemite National Park, with 3.5 million visitors, didn't draw many more people. But despite the numbers, don't expect the same crowds here that you'll find at Yosemite. Sonoma Coast's visitors tend to come for only hours rather than days, and when they arrive, they can spread out across 17 miles of cliffs, coves, and beaches. And while the great majority of Yosemite's visitors arrive at the height of summer, Sonoma Coast's are likely to come any time of year.

There is much to do at the park. Enjoy a picnic on an isolated beach, amidst the roar of the breakers and the screeching of gulls. Study tidepools teeming with life in the shadow of an imposing sea stack. Watch gray whales frolic in the sea as they migrate to the warm waters of Baja. Hike the headlands in spring, when wildflowers are a riot of color.

One thing you won't want to do, though, is swim in the ocean. The frigid waters and strong rip currents make for a dangerous surf. This is also a breeding area for great white sharks, and they have been known to occasionally attack surfers and divers.

Not all the park is centered on the sea. The secluded Willow Creek area in Pomo Canyon, 3 miles inland, is a lush grassland surrounded by dense forest. Here you can observe wildlife, hike an old Indian trading path to the coast, or simply find relaxing solitude.

There are two developed campgrounds within the park—at Bodega Dunes and at Wright's Beach. In addition, Willow Creek and Pomo Canyon Environmental Campgrounds offer hike-in campsites for a primitive, "get-away-from-it-all" experience. Bodega Head and most beaches are currently open 24 hours a day, although the parks department is considering restricting the hours to reduce crime. Camping is permitted only within the campgrounds. South Salmon Creek Beach, Bodega Dunes, Wright's Beach, and Russian Gulch are day-use areas only.

Sonoma Coast State Park Facilities and Activities

	Facilities											Activities										
	Fee Area	Camping - Developed	Camping - Environmental	Restrooms	Showers	Trailer Sanitary Station	Telephone	Picnic Area	Visitor Center	Beach Access	Disabled Access	Hiking	Horseback Riding	Mountain Biking (Paved Roads Only)	Tidepooling	Whale Watching	Seal Watching	Fishing	Rock Climbing	Surfing	Scuba Diving/Snorkeling	Sea Kayaking
Bodega Head				●				●		●	●	●			●	●		●	●		●	
Campbell Cove				●				●		●		●						●				●
Bodega Dunes	●	●		●	●	●	●	●		●	●	●	●					●		●		
South Salmon Creek Beach				●				●		●		●						●		●		●
North Salmon Creek Beach				●				●		●						●		●		●		●
Miwok Beach										●						●		●				
Coleman Beach										●					●	●		●				
Arched Rock Beach										●					●	●		●				
Marshall Gulch										●					●	●		●			●	
Carmet Beach										●					●	●		●			●	
Schoolhouse Beach				●				●		●					●	●		●				
Portuguese Beach				●				●		●					●	●		●				
Gleason Beach																●						
Rock Point								●										●				
Duncans Landing								●		●						●		●				●
Wrights Beach	●	●		●			●	●		●	●	●				●		●				
Furlong Gulch										●		●				●		●			●	●
Shell Beach				●						●		●			●	●		●	●	●	●	
Blind Beach				●						●		●				●		●		●	●	●
Goat Rock Beach				●				●		●							●	●		●		●
Jenner/Jenner Beach				●			●	●	●	●							●	●		●	●	●
Russian Gulch				●				●		●		●						●			●	●
Willow Creek	●		●	●				●		●		●						●				
Pomo Canyon	●		●	●				●				●										
Vista Point				●				●		●	●	●										
Red Hill												●										

First acquired by the State in 1934, Sonoma Coast's boundaries have been expanded several times. A few stretches of private land still lie interspersed among State properties, so watch for signs and don't trespass, especially near Portuguese Beach, Gleason Beach, Shell Beach, and Duncan's Landing.

Historically, Sonoma Coast has been at the forefront of the environmental battleground. For much of the 1960s, a dedicated band waged a protracted and eventually successful battle to stop a nuclear power plant from being built at Bodega Head. In 1972 another battle was waged and won to prevent subdivisions from being built just north of Wright's Beach. Evidence of this fight remains today in the form of a few deserted roads and three houses now owned by the State.

Originally designated a State Beach and intended primarily to provide recreational opportunities, ongoing land acquisitions have continually expanded the park's borders. It now includes significant natural and cultural areas well inland. In 2007, Sonoma Coast was reclassified as a State Park, giving it a legal ability to preserve these resources that would not be possible as a state beach.

Getting There

There are two main routes to the park. To reach the southern portion, take Bodega Highway west from Sebastopol to its intersection with State Highway 1. Go north 4 miles to the town of Bodega Bay. All beaches except Bodega Head are accessible directly from the highway north of town. To reach Bodega Head, turn left at Eastshore Road on the north side of town, turn right at the stop sign, and follow the road to its end.

Another route to the park's northern region is west out of Guerneville via State Highway 116. When you reach State Highway 1 just south of Jenner, you have two choices. Turn right to reach the Jenner Visitor's Center and coastal access points in Jenner and at Russian Gulch. Turn left and cross the Russian River at Bridgehaven for the beaches at Goat Rock, Shell Beach, and all points south. This is also the way to Willow Creek—from Highway 1, turn left on Willow Creek Road immediately after crossing the Russian River highway bridge.

If you're up for a little adventure, Coleman Valley Road offers breathtaking views of the coast. This narrow, winding road out of Occidental was once voted the most scenic drive in Sonoma County. It is little more than one lane wide for much of its length, making it unsuitable for recreational vehicles or vehicles with trailers. The road reaches Highway 1 just north of Coleman Beach. Save this drive for a clear day when you can clearly see the spectacular coastline. A tip: you'll better appreciate the views by driving toward the ocean rather than away from it.

Natural Environment

You can think of Sonoma Coast State Park as four distinct regions: Bodega Head, Bodega Dunes, the northern coast, and the Willow Creek area. Each has a distinct natural environment. Bodega Head is an exposed, brush-covered, rocky headland, while Bodega Dunes has some of the most expansive sand dunes in the State. The coast north of Bodega Bay alternates between sandy beaches and rocky bluffs, while the Willow Creek area consists of grasslands surrounded by dense forest.

Bodega Head

The erosion-resistant granite of Bodega Head stands in stark contrast to the marine sediments lying east of the harbor. Separated by the San Andreas Fault, its rocks are geologically unrelated to those inland. Over the last 30 million years the Head has moved hundreds of miles northward. It now stands as the last exposure of granitic basement rock along the coast north of San Francisco. Other exposures include Point Reyes and the Farallon Islands.

One weekend each April, Bodega Bay celebrates the annual Fisherman's Festival. Two days of celebration include barbeques, live music, bathtub races, and a fine-arts show and crafts fair. Events culminate in a parade of colorfully decorated fishing boats and the blessing of the fleet by local clergymen. Bodega Head is a popular spot to watch the festivities. Crowds can be enormous, so get there early for a good spot. For more information, call the Sonoma Coast Visitor's Center in Bodega Bay at 707-875-3866, or check online at www.bodegabay.com.

Directions

Take Highway 1 to the north side of Bodega Bay. Turn west at the large sign labeled BODEGA HEAD–WESTSIDE PARK–MARINAS at Eastshore Road. Follow the road down the hill and turn right at the stop sign. This is Bay Flat Road, which becomes Westshore Road at a large dirt parking area on the right. (If you have horses, you can park here and ride the trail to Bodega Dunes.) Campbell Cove sits at the southern end of the road, 3 miles from the stop sign. To reach the rocky headlands, continue around the hairpin turn sharply right and up the hill. Bodega Head is open 24 hours but no overnight camping is allowed.

Campbell Cove

It's hard to imagine any sane person wanting to build a nuclear power plant atop the San Andreas Fault, but that's exactly what the Pacific Gas and Electric Company once tried to do at Campbell Cove. In 1958, without any public hearings, they began construction. The outraged citizens of Bodega Bay, led by the feisty Rose Gaffney, immediately rallied to stop the work. The ensuing legal battles lasted a decade, but sanity eventually prevailed. Today, the only remaining evidence of this aborted project is a water-filled excavation pit known as Hole-in-the-Head.

Campbell Cove has recently emerged as a credible contender for the site of Sir Francis Drake's landfall in 1579. Author Brian Kelleher, in his well-researched book, *Drake's Bay*, has cited a number of convincing arguments, including the quality of its harbor, its match to Drake's recorded latitude, and the fact that the surrounding land is similar to his description of the landing site. Unfortunately, excavation work for the nuclear power plant probably destroyed any remaining archeological evidence, so scholars will undoubtedly continue to argue these points for decades to come.

Campbell Cove is a favorite spot for families with small children.

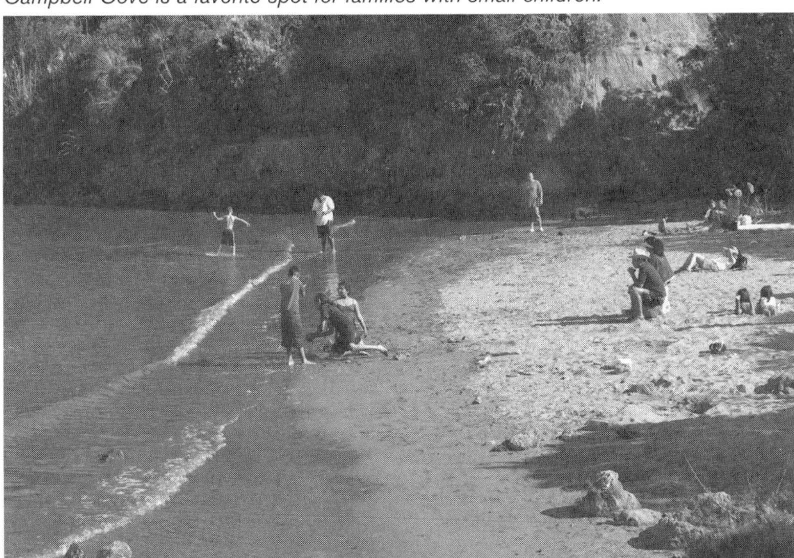

Campbell Cove has a large dirt parking lot, picnic tables, and a wooden outhouse. Its sheltered, sandy beach is perfect for families. At low tide, the mudflats here are an excellent spot for catching crabs or digging clams (a California fishing license is required for anyone age 16 years and older).

Headlands Area

After Campbell Cove, the road winds 0.4 mile to a Y intersection. The right fork leads to the west parking lot overlooking the Pacific. The left fork leads to the east parking lot overlooking the harbor. Cinderblock outhouses are located at both parking lots, but neither has picnic tables.

In winter and early spring, the west lot is a favorite spot for gray whale watching. The southern migration in December and January tends to occur some distance off shore, so the best sightings usually occur during the more leisurely northern migration from February through April. On weekends during the season, volunteers from the Stewards of the Coast and Redwoods are available to help watch for spouts, answer questions about the migration, and discuss the natural history of the whale.

From December through April, Bodega Head is a good spot to watch for gray whales as they migrate along the coast. On most weekend afternoons, volunteers from the Stewards of the Coast and Redwoods are present to help visitors learn more about the whales as they watch for telltale spouts.

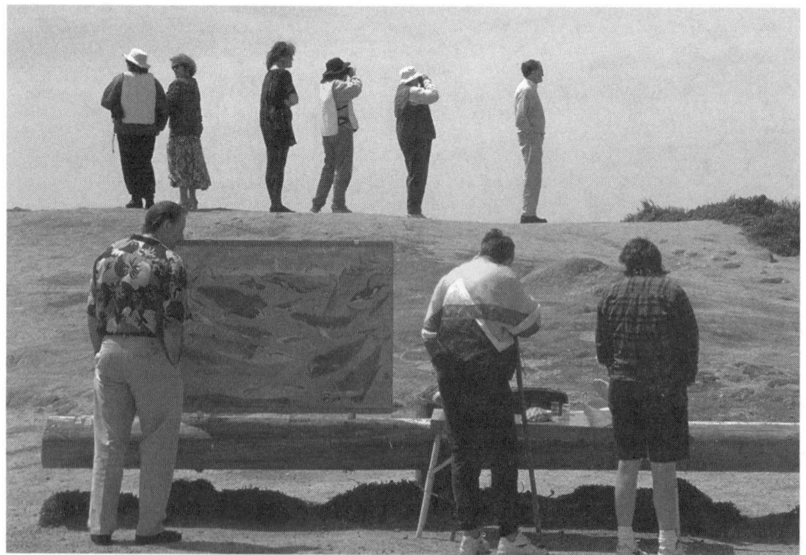

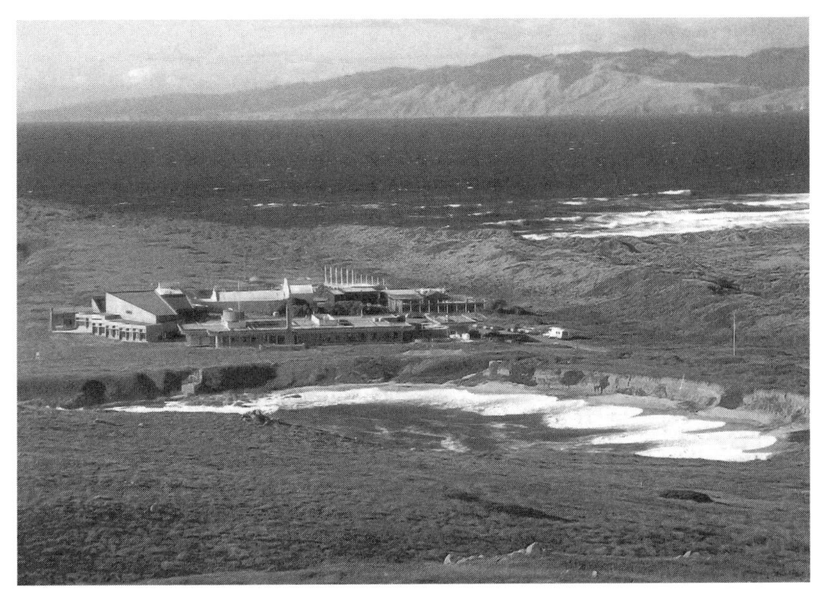

Bodega Marine Reserve. Horseshoe Cove is in the foreground.

A short path at the north end of the west parking lot leads down to a nice little sandy beach at Windmill Cove. The cliffs along the path provide an interesting lesson in geology. The granite-like rock is quartz diorite, overlain by layers of coarse sandstone uplifted from the ocean floor. Look closely at the very top layer of dirt. The dark soil and fragments of seashells suggest this is a former Native American midden. The careful observer might also notice bits of carbonized wood within the soil, estimated to be as much as 40,000 years old.

Bodega Head Hiking Trails

Two main hiking trails branch out from the parking lots at the Head. The Bodega Head Loop winds around the rocky headlands while the Overlook Trail stretches from the Head to South Salmon Creek Beach. Both offer breathtaking views of the coast and, in spring and summer, a profusion of colorful wildflowers. For much of their lengths they are exposed as they traverse the headlands, so save these hikes for a clear day when winds aren't too strong. Neither trail is open to horses or mountain bikes. See the Hiking Trails section beginning on Page 52 for detailed descriptions of these and other Sonoma Coast trails.

Bodega Dunes

Just north of Bodega Head are the sands of Bodega Dunes. These expansive dunes stretch from Bodega Harbor to Salmon Creek, rising as high as 200 feet above the sea. With luck, you may see several of the many species of mammals that reside here, including jackrabbits, voles, mice, badgers, raccoons, and foxes.

Cattle heavily overgrazed the dunes in the late 1800s, almost completely stripping them of vegetation. Without the stabilizing influence of native plants, the sand began shifting and eventually threatened Bodega Harbor. In 1951 a dune stabilization project was started. Various specialized grasses were planted to help keep drifting sands from silting up the harbor. Even today the restoration is not complete, so stay off the sand in fenced-off areas.

Both a campground and a day-use area are located at Bodega Dunes. Because of the extreme danger, no fires are permitted in the dunes.

Directions

The easiest way to the dunes is via the Bodega Dunes Campground road. From Highway 1, turn west at the sign marking the campground. Pay your entrance fee at the kiosk 0.4 mile west of the highway. You can then turn right and go 0.8 mile to the day use parking area or proceed ahead to the campground.

You can also reach the northernmost dunes from the hamlet of Salmon Creek. Follow the directions on Page 34 for South Salmon Creek Beach and walk the boardwalk across the dunes. Stay on the path and avoid the fenced-off dune restoration areas.

Campground

The campground is situated well back from the beach, sheltered by the dunes and stands of eucalyptus and cypress. Three loop roads contain a total of 98 campsites. The upper campground, sites 1–21, backs up to a eucalyptus grove that is home to thousands of monarch butterflies for a short period each fall. Facilities include restrooms with flush toilets, running water, hot showers (the only ones in the park), picnic tables, and a trailer sanitation dump. Reservations are accepted all year through the state park reservation service at 1-800-444-7275, and are strongly advised in the summer.

Day-Use Area

From the day-use parking lot it is only a short hike over low dunes to South Salmon Creek Beach. Until January 2006, a wheelchair-accessible wooden boardwalk made the trek easier, but a strong storm that month destroyed much of it. Although the parks department intends to make repairs, no timetable has yet been set. For now, you will need to walk in the soft sand beside the closed structure.

Various trails extend along the shore and up into the grass- and ice plant-covered dunes. If you hike all the way to Mussel Point at the south end of the beach, remember that the point itself is part of the private Bodega Marine Reserve and is closed to public access.

The picnic area is disabled accessible. It includes numerous tables, several metal fire rings, elevated barbecues, and two wooden outhouses. There is no running water. The picnic area is separated from the beach by a line of dunes and is reasonably protected from wind.

Equestrian Access

The northern part of the beach is reserved for foot traffic, so if you have horses, you need to approach the dunes from the west side off Bay Flat Road. There is a free parking area for horse trailers 0.3 mile west of the junction with Eastshore Road. Horses are permitted on Salmon Creek Beach only up to the boardwalk, which although now closed, is still visible. No dogs are allowed on the trail.

Equestrians ride along South Salmon Creek Beach. Horses must stay south of the boardwalk.

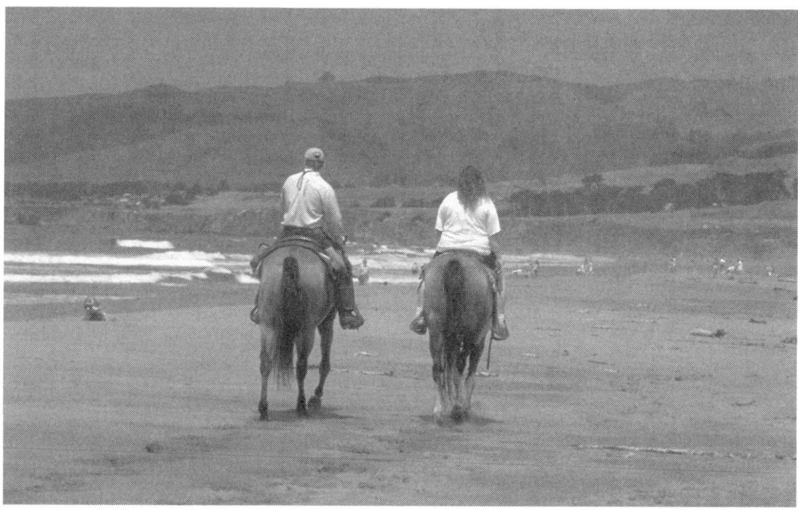

Trails

A number of trails wind throughout the dunes, which are broader and higher than they might first seem. It is easy to get lost, and while you are unlikely to be in any real danger, you may find yourself taking a much longer hike than you anticipated. Detailed trail descriptions begin on Page 52.

Northern Coast

The most popular part of the park runs from Salmon Creek north past the mouth of the Russian River. Highway 1 runs right along the edge of the bluffs here, giving you easy beach access at numerous points. The more popular beaches tend to have large parking lots and reasonably easy trails. Some spots have narrow trails that cling precariously to the cliff sides, while a few have only the faintest hint of a trail. Use common sense and don't try to descend unless you're sure it is safe. Remember that the coast is unforgiving, and a moment of carelessness could have tragic consequences.

For most of this distance, the park extends from Highway 1 to the sea, but there are still several stretches of private property interspersed along the way. These include the land between Portuguese Beach and Gleason Beach, at Rock Point, at Ocean View, and the houses on the bluff above Goat Rock. Don't trespass in these areas.

South Salmon Creek Beach

This broad, sandy beach, flanked by Bodega Dunes, is a favorite spot for surfers. It extends over 2 miles from Salmon Creek south to Mussel Point. The most northerly access is by way of Bean Avenue in the hamlet of Salmon Creek. The parking lot at the end of the road is usually full on nice days, especially on weekend afternoons.

You won't see any indication of beach access from the highway, so watch for the turn-off just south of the Salmon Creek Bridge at milepost 12.41. The narrow road meanders through a residential area reminiscent of a New England fishing village. Keep to the right, staying on Bean Avenue, and drive all the way to the free parking lot at the end of the road. From 7 P.M. Friday to 6 A.M. Monday, parking is not allowed on the road until you reach this parking lot on state park property. From here, hike over a broad expanse of grass-covered dunes to the beach.

North Salmon Creek Beach

This is one of the most popular spots along the entire Sonoma Coast. It has plenty of free parking, easy coastal access, and a long sandy beach that's great for picnicking, kite flying, Frisbee throwing, and surf fishing. On hot summer weekends parking is at a premium, and this beach can resemble the crowded ones of Southern California. Even in winter you'll rarely be alone—I counted over two dozen people here on a cold December afternoon with storm seas raging and angry clouds threatening a deluge at any moment. At any time of year you are likely to see wetsuit-clad surfers riding the waves here.

Several parking areas dot this stretch of the highway. Some are paved, some are just gravel pullouts at the side of the road. The best is a large paved lot just north of milepost 12.75. It has two wooden outhouse buildings on its east side, but no running water. A paved trail from the restrooms leads down to the Salmon Creek estuary. When the creek mouth silts up, it forms a broad lagoon that is a favorite roost for a variety of shorebirds. Some of the species you may see include gulls, herons, egrets, sandpipers, loons, and pelicans. There is an easy trail at the west end of this lot leading directly to the beach 30 feet below.

On a warm summer day, South Salmon Creek Beach can resemble the crowded beaches of Southern California. The surf can be treacherous even on hot days, so always observe the rules of ocean safety on Page 18.

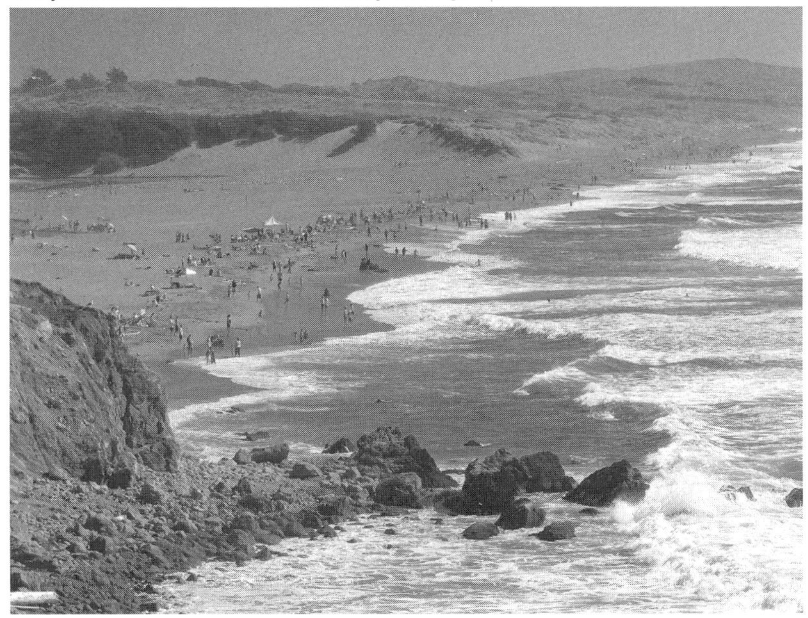

Miwok Beach

This pleasant sandy beach is named after the Miwok Indians that originally inhabited the southern Sonoma Coast. Its small parking area, just large enough for four cars, is well marked and directly adjacent to the highway. You won't find any restrooms here. A steep, partially paved trail leads 60 feet down to the beach. Stone steps at the bottom of the trail simplify access to the beach.

The southern edge of Miwok Beach merges with North Salmon Creek Beach. At low tide you can easily walk the full distance to Salmon Creek, but the beach shrinks considerably at high tide.

Coleman Beach

The parking area at this beach is a small paved lot just south of highway milepost 13.46. A narrow asphalt trail once descended the side of the cliff, but it has now eroded away and is closed. It will eventually be rebuilt as funds permit.

At low tide you may be able to reach this beach by hiking north from Salmon Creek. Look for a scenic waterfall cascading down the cliff north of this beach after seasonal rains.

Arched Rock Beach

A large parking lot on a bluff directly off the highway provides excellent views of the rocky coast to the north and Salmon Creek Beach to the south. A very poor trail, not maintained by the State, leads part way down the cliff, but heavy rains in February 1998, the wettest month

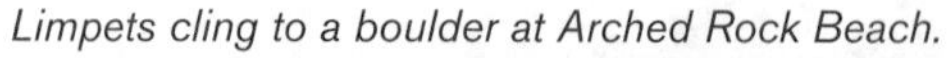

Limpets cling to a boulder at Arched Rock Beach.

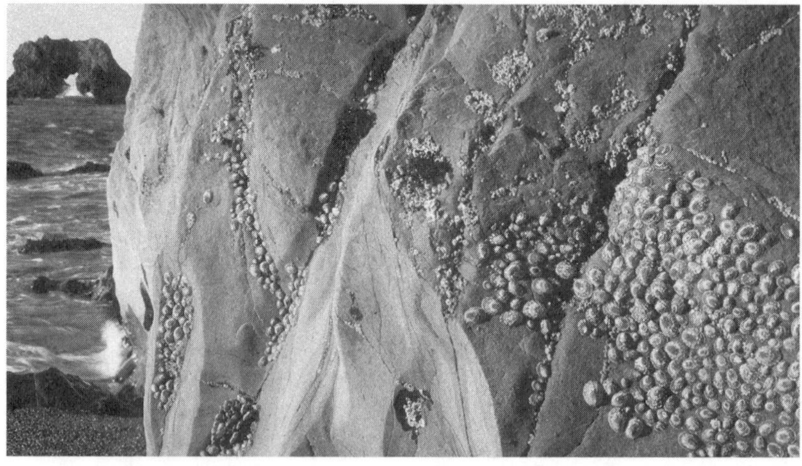

in Sonoma County history, nearly obliterated the bottom half. If you really want to ignore common sense and scramble down to this beach, wear hiking boots or good athletic shoes, use your hands and knees to pick your way down the loose cliffs, and don't blame me if you fall and break your neck. Once down, you'll find a small isolated beach consisting of polished, multicolored pea gravel. The namesake rock, an offshore sea stack with a hole in the middle, is visible a few hundred yards to the north. (Note that this is not the same Arched Rock that is prominent farther north near Blind Beach.) This beach is nearly gone at high tide, so keep track of the tide if you decide to descend. There are no restrooms at this beach.

Marshall Gulch

You'll find a sheltered, sandy beach (nearly obscured at high tide) on the south side of the gulch. The rocky north side nominally connects to Carmet Beach, but hiking over the slippery rocks is difficult and dangerous even at low tide. There is a small, paved parking area on a bluff just north of the gulch. Arched Rock lies directly west, but because of its angle, you can't see the arch from here. A good but narrow gravel trail leads from the south end of the parking lot down to the beach.

Carmet Beach

Two trails from this large parking area lead 40 feet down to beaches. A good but steep trail on the south side leads right down to a small sandy beach. Another less well-maintained trail on the north side leads to a somewhat larger sandy beach with a rocky surfline. You'll see much evidence of crumbling cliffs at the base of this beach. These are good spots for tidepooling.

Schoolhouse Beach

A large parking lot here can hold dozens of cars in a sort of free-for-all arrangement. The deep, isolated beach lies to the north of the lot. A wide access road (closed to vehicles) leads down to the coarse gravel beach. A dual wooden outhouse sits halfway down the road. This is a favorite spot for walking dogs (remember to keep Fido on a leash at all times).

Portuguese Beach

This popular sandy beach is about half a mile long and deep enough that it is still accessible even at high tide. The large parking area is on a bluff at the south side of the beach. Two trails lead down to the beach. The one closest to the highway is a very easy, wide gravel road that ends high up on the sand. A wooden outhouse is located here. The more westerly trail is much steeper, with switchbacks and many steps, but ends right at the surf. In fact, the last several wooden steps are held by wire cables designed to let them float at high tide.

Gleason Beach

A sign proclaiming Gleason Beach marks this small parking lot on a bluff 50 feet above the ocean, but don't expect to reach the beach here. An old trail at the south end of the lot has long since eroded away and is not scheduled to be repaired. Don't try to climb down to the beach here. Instead, stay in the parking lot, enjoy the views, and admire the large sea stack directly across from you.

Rock Point

This is a good spot for a short rest to relax and view the rugged coastline. A gravel parking lot well off the highway provides excellent views of the rocky shoreline. There are no restrooms and no beach access from here. Please respect the private property at the north end of this lot.

Duncan's Cove

A moderately large parking area here includes two picnic tables with great views of the coast. A steep but well-maintained trail at the north side of the lot leads down to Duncan's Cove 50 feet below. There are no restrooms at this beach.

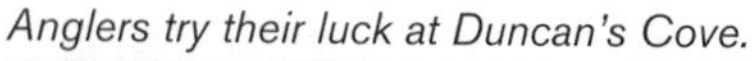

Anglers try their luck at Duncan's Cove.

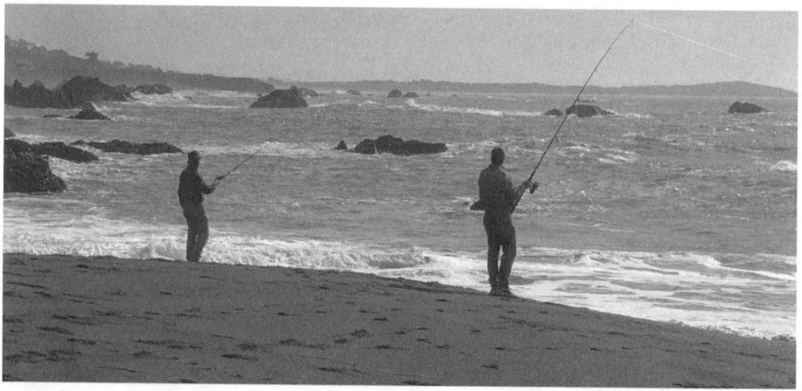

Duncan's Landing

This rocky promontory shelters a cove that was once a doghole port for lumber schooners. Wright's Beach is to the north and Duncan's Cove to the south. From 1862 to 1877, Samuel and Alexander Duncan used a horse-drawn railway to deliver lumber to the landing from their mill at Bridgehaven on the Russian River. Schooners were loaded using a wooden slide chute that extended down from the cliff.

Eventually, the narrow-gauge railroad pushed through from Occidental to the Russian River, so the Duncan brothers moved to the present site of Duncans Mills and shipped their lumber by rail. After that, the port was still used to ship such staples as butter, potatoes, and vegetables. During Prohibition, it was a favorite anchorage for rumrunners.

A short, paved access road leads from the highway to the rocky point. There it becomes a one-way loop with several parking areas, some with picnic tables. A good trail at the north end of the loop leads 60 feet down to Wright's Beach. Directly off the point are two large sea stacks—an onshore stack called the Hogback and an island known as Death Rock. It didn't come by that name accidentally, for Death Rock

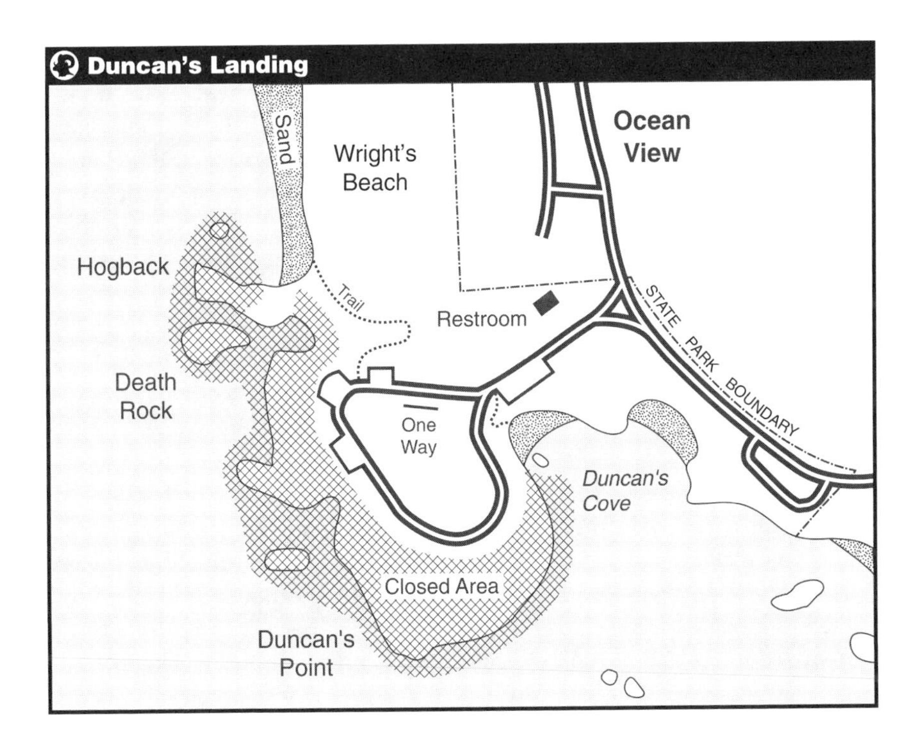

is one of the most deadly spots along the entire California coast. Even though the entire shoreline around Duncan's Landing, including Death Rock, is closed to public access, it still manages to claim at least one victim nearly every year as people ignore the warnings and scramble up the rock, only to be washed away by rogue waves.

Along the south side of the access road is another parking area and trail down to Duncan's Cove. A cinderblock restroom, partially hidden by trees across the road from this trailhead, is closed indefinitely.

Wright's Beach

This popular beach consists of a picnic area and campground at the end of a short paved road winding down to the beach. Restrooms in the campground provide running water and flush toilets but no showers. Both the beach and the restrooms are wheelchair accessible.

This is one of the few spots in the park where day-use fees are presently collected. The parking area and picnic tables lie directly back from the beach, buffered by a low ridge of dune grass. The wide, sandy beach stretches for over a mile and is popular with fishermen, divers, and beachcombers. Obey posted signs and stay away from Death Rock at the south end of the beach.

The 30-site Wright's Beach Campground lies north of the parking lot, partially protected by trees and shrubs. Campsites are closely spaced but separated by bushes to give some sense of privacy. The more northerly sites back directly up to the beach. It is a pleasant enough campground on a calm day, but when the wind picks up you'll be happier in the confines of an RV rather than being buffeted in a tent. The campground, designated as "premium" by the park system, is on the reservation system all year. Reservations are strongly advised during the summer. Call the state park reservation service at 1-800-444-7275, to reserve a campsite.

Wright's Beach is the southern terminus of the Kortum Trail, a 4-mile-long seaside path along the headlands that starts near Goat Rock.

Furlong Gulch

You won't see a parking area anywhere near Furlong Gulch, or even a road sign to mark its presence, but if you know how to get there, you'll find an excellent isolated beach surrounded by high bluffs. When I was there one sunny winter afternoon there wasn't another soul in site, not even footprints on the coarse dark sand. It's the perfect spot for getting away from it all. (But don't expect isolation on a summer weekend!)

The Kortum Trail crosses here barely 50 feet from the beach, so you can park at Shell Beach and make an easy half-mile hike south to the gulch. The wildflowers along this trail can be spectacular in the spring. But beware—during the rainy season the gulch can be an impassible torrent of water.

An even easier access is from the south. Drive to milepost 17.65 and turn west on Carlevaro Way, part of an abandoned subdivision now owned by the State. The two houses to the south are homes for state park staff. Don't disturb the residents; instead, turn right onto Grill Way and park at the end of the road. From here, a path leads west a short distance to connect with the Kortum Trail. Hike north a few hundred feet until the trail descends the side of the gully, then head west to the beach.

Shell Beach

If your interest leans toward beachcombing and tidepool exploration, this is the spot to go. The rocky north end nurtures a host of marine life and is frequently used by elementary schools as an outdoor classroom. There is also a sandy beach to the south that is popular for fishing and picnicking. It is also a geological wonder, an excellent example of a subduction zone (see sidebar on page 42).

From the large Shell Beach sign on the highway, follow a short paved road to a large parking lot with a dual wooden outhouse at its west end. From here, a 500-foot-long trail winds down the bluff to the beach. The steep trail includes numerous wooden steps as you descend, including a series of planks on cables all the way to the beach.

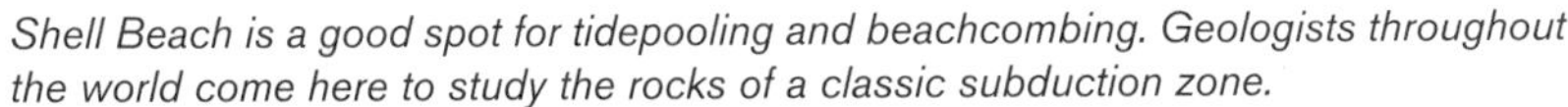
Shell Beach is a good spot for tidepooling and beachcombing. Geologists throughout the world come here to study the rocks of a classic subduction zone.

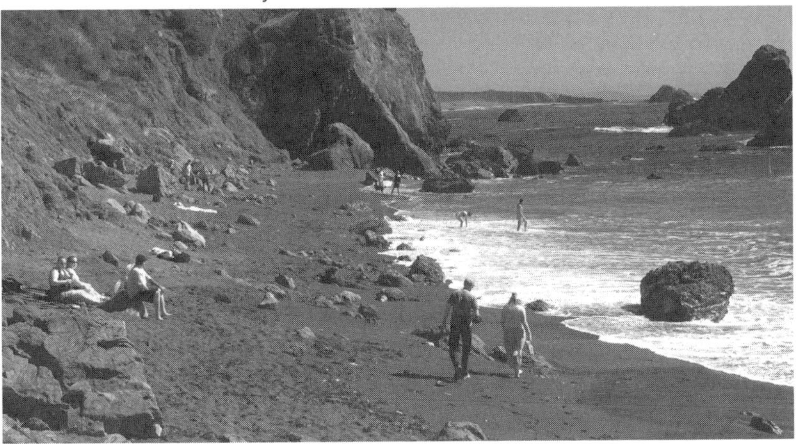

The tidepools are best explored at low tide, so check a local newspaper or consult a tide table before your trip. You can also check online data for the Bodega Harbor Entrance at www.tidesonline.com.

At Shell Beach, use caution when climbing over the slippery, algae-covered rocks. Be sure to obey the rules of ocean safety listed on Page 18 and review the section on intertidal life on Page 17. Some of the organisms found here include limpets, mussels, turban snails, anemones, sea stars, chitons, sea urchins, hermit crabs, and shore crabs. Remember that tidepool life is protected within the park, so try to return anything you pick up (including rocks with sea life attached) to the exact position you found it. Fishermen need a valid California sport fishing license in their

Shell Beach Geology

Long before the formation of the San Andreas Fault, the land around Shell Beach was a scene of great geologic activity. According to the theory of plate tectonics described in Chapter 1, the earth is comprised of a series of rigid plates that ride on top of a more fluid mantle, much like ice floating on water. The reason the San Francisco Bay Area sees so many earthquakes is because it lies where two plates are colliding–the North American Plate to the east and the Pacific Plate to the west. But 100 million years ago this collision had not yet begun. At that time, the North American Plate was sliding over the top of another eastward-moving oceanic plate, the Farallon Plate. The immense weight of the North American Plate pushed the edge of the Farallon Plate far down into the earth's mantle, where heat and pressure transformed the chemical composition of its rock through a process called metamorphism.

The junction where one tectonic plate slides over another is called a *subduction zone*. As the North American Plate scraped across the top of the Farallon Plate like a bulldozer pushing dirt, a wedge of rocks called a *mélange* accumulated in the subduction zone. The land around Shell Beach is part of this mélange, a rock assemblage known as the Franciscan Complex. Now raised above sea level, rocks of the Franciscan Complex are found throughout the Bay Area. These rocks are typical of the many types found in a subduction zone. They include the metamorphic rocks peridotite, serpentine, greenstone, blueschist, and eclogite, the sedimentary rocks chert, shale, and greywacke sandstone, and the igneous rock known as pillow lava, all mixed chaotically together. Shell Beach offers an outstanding opportunity to see a full cross-section of this mélange by way of an easy walk.

Start from the Shell Beach parking lot and hike the trail down to the beach. As you walk, study the surrounding rocks. Two blue-gray boulders with dark streaks near the top of the bluff on your left are blueschist, a metamorphic rock rich in the mineral glaucophane. Blueschist is formed when volcanic basalt is subjected to heat and pressure in a subduction zone.

possession and may only take those species designated in the current California Sport Fishing Regulations.

Blind Beach

Yet another long sandy beach, this one is a good spot for smelt fishing, beachcombing, and solitary strolls. The northern end adjacent to the Goat Rock parking lot is easily accessed and therefore more heavily visited. If you're looking for more solitude and don't mind a hike, you should enter from the Blind Beach parking lot, 0.75 mile down Goat Rock Road. The trail meanders 0.5 mile down to the southern end of the beach 200 feet below (be careful—poison oak grows profusely along the

Continuing down the trail, you reach a creekbed on your left with boulders of serpentine, a blue-green metamorphic rock created by the reaction of seawater with olivine. Take a closer look at these rocks and you will see scraped and polished surfaces caused by extreme pressure exerted on them in the depths of the subduction zone.

At the beach, a smorgasbord of rocks lies scattered about, including graywacke sandstone, peridotite, and greenstone. In the sand near the trailhead, look for a massive gray-green rock with bulbous pillow-like shapes across its surface. This is pillow lava, formed when molten basalt erupts under the sea and is quickly cooled. Other pillow lavas can be found in the bluffs near Blind Beach.

At the base of the cliff just north of the trailhead is a dark-orange layered rock that is an excellent example of chert, a silica-rich rock from deep in the ocean. Since silica is not abundant in seawater, no one knows exactly how chert forms. Silica-based microorganisms called radiolaria do live in the oceans, and one theory suggests they become especially abundant when volcanic activity deposits silica-rich ash into the sea. When the vulcanism stops, the radiolaria die and sink to the seafloor, forming a layer of chert that is soon covered by mud washed down from the land. Eventually the vulcanism resumes and the radiolaria bloom again. This cycle, repeated over and over, lays down layer after layer of chert separated by mud. The sample at Shell Beach, with its bent and folded layers, graphically illustrates this alternating sequence of chert and mudstone repeated numerous times.

About 10 million years ago, the Shell Beach subduction zone ceased to exist as the Farallon Plate, pushed along by the eastward moving Pacific Plate, was completely consumed under the North American Plate. Yet the Farallon Plate may not be gone even today. Many geologists believe it is still scraping along under the North American Plate, causing an occasional earthquake in the Midwest and creating the Basin and Range topography of the western United States as it goes.

trailside). In spring and summer, many wildflowers bloom along this trail. A pair of cinderblock outhouses sits at the north end of the parking lot next to the trailhead.

Goat Rock Beach

This is one of the most popular spots in the park. Goat Rock boasts long sandy beaches, two parking lots, and a picnic area with fire rings. At the extreme north end of the beach you'll usually find a colony of harbor seals lounging lazily on the sand. On weekends, volunteers from the Stewards of the Coast and Redwoods are on hand with binoculars and spotting scopes to help you safely observe them. They can also answer many questions about the seals and their habitat.

Female seals give birth to pups between March and June. A pup sometimes appears to be abandoned, but don't worry. It has generally been left behind only temporarily while the mother forages for food. Keep your distance—not only is it against the law to harass the seals,

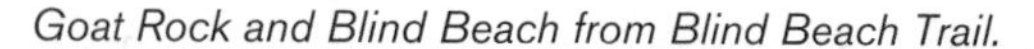

Goat Rock and Blind Beach from Blind Beach Trail.

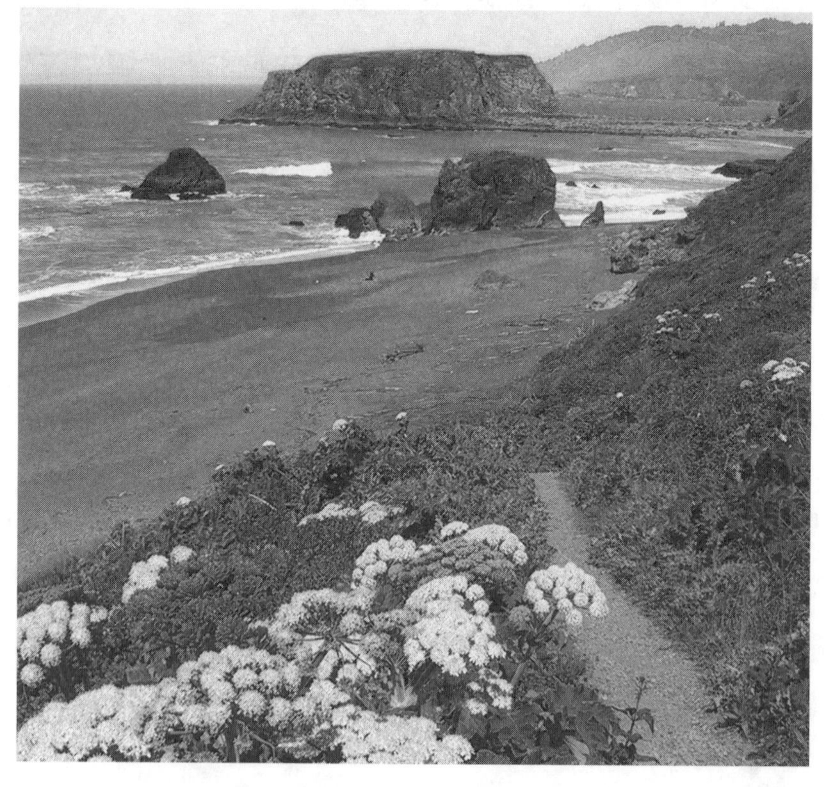

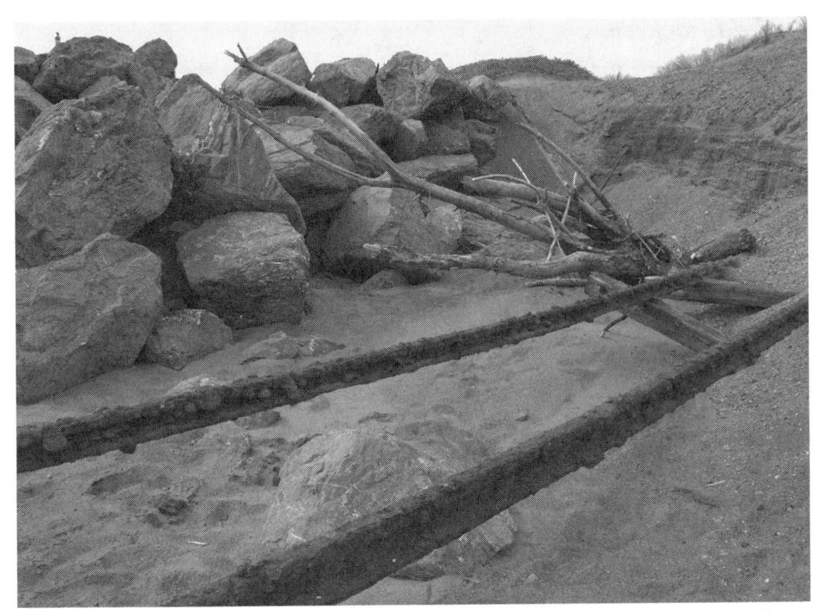

In the early 20th century, countless tons of rocks were hauled over these railroad tracks at Goat Rock Beach to help build a breakwater at the mouth of the Russian River. The breakwater was washed away after only a few years, but remnants of the tracks remain.

you'll find that both adults and pups can inflict serious bites. A raised head can be a signal of alarm and distress for a seal, not always mere curiosity.

Goat Rock itself looks like an enormous sea stack, but until the 1920s it was actually a peninsula. Rock from the bluff was quarried down to the height of the current parking lot to help form a breakwater at the mouth of the Russian River. You can still see remnants of the concrete breakwater on the north end of Goat Rock Beach, as well as the rusted remains of the railway used to haul the rock.

To reach Goat Rock Beach, turn west from Highway 1 at the large wooden sign near milepost 19.15. Follow the road to its end, where it branches in two directions. The left fork leads to the north end of Blind Beach and to Goat Rock, named for the herds of goats that lived here while it was still a peninsula. The parking lot here extends from shore all the way to the rock. (For safety reasons, Goat Rock itself is closed to the public.)

The right fork leads down to the beach parking lot and picnic area. There are metal fire rings here for picnickers. It is only a short hike over low dunes to the beach, but a good 500 yards north to the seal colony.

Arched Rock View

In the water off Blind Beach is an enormous sea stack with a huge hole in it. Called Arched Rock on maps, it is much larger than the rock to the south for which Arched Rock Beach is named. In fact it is so large that intrepid kayakers have been known to paddle through it when seas are calm—not something to be recommended here, however.

The Arched Rock View parking area, 1.25 miles down Goat Rock Road, gives you an excellent view of this geologic wonder.

Jenner

Stop at the Jenner Visitor Center for the latest information on park activities, seal and whale activity, and general information on the coast. You'll also find a number of books, postcards, and clothing related to the coast. The center, open weekends from 10–4 (subject to availability

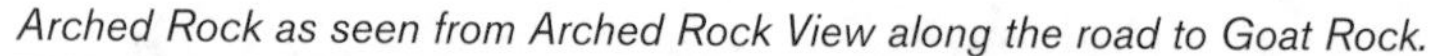

Arched Rock as seen from Arched Rock View along the road to Goat Rock.

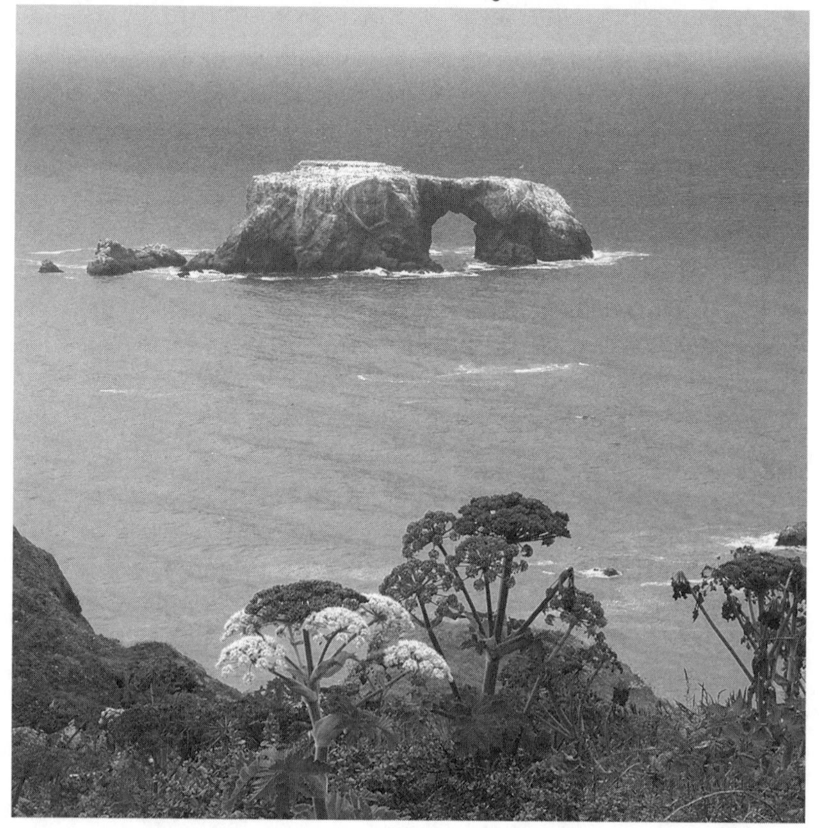

of volunteers), is located in a historic former boathouse directly across the road from the service station/convenience store. John Easdale, a renowned boat builder, made beautifully crafted canoes and rowboats here in the 1930s and 40s.

There are several coastal access points just north of town. The most popular trail leads from a small dirt parking area just north of milepost 22.24. Hike 80 feet down the moderately steep trail to a long, sandy beach on the north side of the Russian River. You can get an excellent view of the seal colony—usually across the river, but sometimes on this side. Remember to stay back approximately 50 feet and do not disturb the animals. If they are raising their heads you are too close.

For a panoramic view of the coast, stop at one of the two dirt pullouts near milepost 22.53. If you are reasonably athletic, you may want to walk to a peak formed by a highway-cut just north of the parking area. From here, follow a narrow, overgrown trail around the west side of the peak and then steeply down. Descend carefully to an exposed granite promontory with spectacular views. Goat Rock Beach and the Russian River mouth lie to the south, while views of the rocky coastline lie to the north. Save this hike for a time when the winds aren't too strong.

Russian Gulch

The parking area for Russian Gulch is just over 2 miles north of Jenner. Watch for the dirt road on the west side of the highway near milepost 24.55. A gate at the entrance closes at sunset or whenever the rangers get around to it. The trail leaves from the end of the lot just past the outhouse. The beach is a 0.2-mile hike through alders, willows, and dense underbrush. In 2007, state park staff and volunteers cleared the worst of the underbrush so that the trail is now reasonably easy to navigate. (You'll still feel a bit like you're walking through a haunted forest in the most overgrown portions of the path.) When you reach the beach, make a mental note of the trail location, as it may not be obvious when you're ready to leave. Tall cliffs on either side shelter the isolated beach. Several picnic tables sit on a sandy bench south of the creek.

Northern Hiking Trails

You'll have impressive views from any of the northern area's three main hiking trails. Kortum Trail and Vista Trail are relatively easy walks, while the Pomo Canyon/Red Hill Trail is more strenuous. Be sure to take along water, snacks, and protection from sun and wind. Horses and mountain bikes are not allowed on any of these trails. You'll find complete trail descriptions beginning on Page 52.

Willow Creek Area

The Willow Creek area lies in a broad canyon well back from the sea, separated by a line of hills. Lower Willow Creek, open to everyone, is accessed from Highway 1. Upper Willow Creek, accessed from Highway 116, is open only to holders of special permits.

The weather in Willow Creek can be vastly different from the nearby coast. While the shoreline is blanketed in fog, Willow Creek may be bathed in sunlight and 15°F warmer. Two environmental campgrounds lie within the lower canyon. Willow Creek Environmental Camp sits on the Russian River, and Pomo Canyon Environmental Camp is 3 miles inland. The Dr. David Joseph Memorial Pomo Canyon Trail, described on Page 72, provides a vigorous hike through redwood forests and open grasslands along a former Indian trading route.

In 2005, the State added an additional 3,373 acres in upper Willow Creek. The State currently lacks funds to operate it, so they have contracted with LandPaths, a local volunteer organization, to manage it. You may only enter upper Willow Creek if you have gone through a training class and have obtained a free permit from LandPaths, or if you are joining a docent-led hike. Details on how to obtain a permit are available on the LandPaths website, www.LandPaths.org.

Islands in the Sky Vista Loop Trail, described on Page 78, is the most popular trail within upper Willow Creek. It offers some of the most spectacular views within the entire park.

Directions

Access to lower Willow Creek is unrestricted. If you're coming from Jenner, take Highway 1 south. Immediately after crossing the Russian River highway bridge, turn east onto Willow Creek Road. If you're coming from Bodega Bay, take Highway 1 north. Willow Creek Road is 0.6 mile past the turnoff for Goat Rock Beach. The Willow Creek Environmental Camp is on your left 0.5 mile from the highway, immediately past a house occupied by state park staff. Pomo Canyon Environmental Camp is down a dirt road on your right, 2.8 miles from the highway.

To reach upper Willow Creek from Santa Rosa, take Highway 101 north to the River Road exit and turn left (west). Follow River Road 15 miles to the town of Guerneville, where it merges with Highway 116. Drive through the town and continue on Highway 116 another 8 miles to the town of Duncans Mills. Turn left at Moscow Road, cross the bridge, and make an immediate right on Freezeout Road. Follow this road about a quarter mile to the second gate on your left. Permit holders may unlock the gate and proceed another quarter mile to the grassy parking area.

Willow Creek Environmental Camp

This is the only state park campground on the Russian River. Eleven primitive sites are available on a first-come-first-serve basis. You must self-register and pay your registration fee at the parking lot, which is a half mile down a dirt road from the junction with Willow Creek Road. The campground is open April 1 to November 30.

Like all environmental camps, Willow Creek is intended to provide a more secluded experience than possible at a developed campground. Sites are widely spaced and located for maximum privacy. Vehicles aren't allowed at the campsites, so you'll have to park in the lot and carry in your equipment. It's an easy walk of 90 to 770 yards, depending on your site. A pit toilet is located nearby.

Most of the sites sit in the trees surrounding a meadow. Site 10 is on the riverbank. All sites have tables and all but site 5, which is located in an area of high fire danger, have metal fire rings. You must bring your own wood for fires, as you are not allowed to gather wood in the state park. Bring your own water, since there is none at the camp and Russian River water is unsuitable for drinking. Pets are not allowed at any environmental camp because wildlife will avoid areas frequented by domesticated animals.

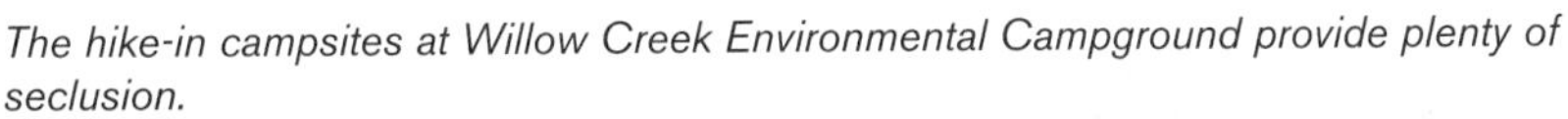

The hike-in campsites at Willow Creek Environmental Campground provide plenty of seclusion.

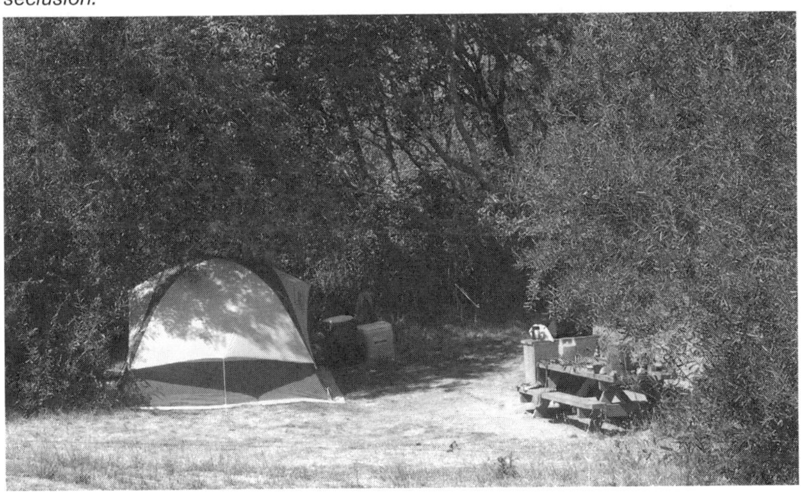

Pomo Canyon Environmental Camp

Like Willow Creek, this campground is designed to give you a sense of solitude. The entrance road stretches 0.4 mile from Willow Creek Road through a grassy meadow to the parking area. The 20 campsites, including one accessible to the disabled, are situated in a redwood grove at the edge of the meadow within 0.3 mile of the parking lot. Once you have picked a site, you must self-register and pay the fee. You must carry your equipment from the lot to your campsite. Two pit toilets stand at the base of the trail, and there is a water spigot near the trailhead. No pets are allowed. The campground is open April 1 through November 30.

Upper Willow Creek

Access to Upper Willow Creek is restricted to people who have taken a training course and received a permit, or individuals who are traveling with permit holders. Louisiana-Pacific Corporation logged Upper Willow Creek for many years before selling it to the Mendocino Redwood Company in 1998. In 2005, the State closed a deal in which 3,373 acres of this tract were purchased with the help of additional funding from the Sonoma County Agricultural Preservation and Open Space District, the California Coastal Conservancy, and the Wildlife Conservation Board. But the State did not have enough money to open the acquisition to the public, so the non-profit organization LandPaths agreed to manage it for at least the first four years. The eventual plan, when funding becomes available, is to open the tract to unrestricted public access.

Access is currently administered through a permit program. Individuals who take a mandatory training course taught by LandPaths are issued permits allowing them to enter the property to hike, bike, or horseback ride on it. Individuals who have not obtained a permit may still gain access by joining a regularly scheduled docent-led hike through the property. For more information, visit the LandPaths web site at www.LandPaths.org.

Preserving Sonoma County's Open Space

The Sonoma County you see today is a balanced mix of urban development and rural countryside, but this wasn't always assured. From 1970 to 1990 the population grew from under 200,000 to more than 450,000 people. Housing developments seemed to spring up overnight, and there was a real danger the county would become an endless sprawl of urbanization like the San Francisco-San Jose corridor to the south.

Residents railed against uncontrolled growth, and in 1990 voters overwhelmingly passed a ballot measure creating the Sonoma County Agricultural and Open Space District, a first-in-the-nation use of tax dollars to acquire and preserve agricultural and open space lands. Funded by a quarter-cent sales tax, the district has protected nearly 75,000 acres–an area over twice the size of Santa Rosa–through conservation agreements and outright purchases. Along the coast, the District helped acquire the Red Hill and Willow Creek properties for Sonoma Coast State Park, and the Wright Hill and Carrington Ranches, planned future additions.

The Open Space District is not alone in preserving Sonoma County's rural environment. The private Sonoma Land Trust has been helping with preservation since 1976. In late 2008, the Trust announced a milestone agreement to purchase 5,630 acres northeast of the town of Jenner. When completed, the Jenner Headlands will be the single largest conservation land acquisition in Sonoma County history. The property's attractions include redwood forests, fish-bearing streams, magnificent coastal views, and an abundance of wildlife. Public access is still several years away.

The Open Space District can use sales tax revenues to acquire and preserve lands, but not to manage or operate them. For parcels intended for public access rather than agricultural use, the District must find others to operate them. When budgets don't allow the land to be added to existing parks, LandPaths, a private non-profit organization, can often help. LandPaths creates ways for people to experience the beauty and value of the land through such activities as building trails, leading school field trips, networking with landowners, and conducting guided tours on lands not otherwise accessible to the public. On the Sonoma Coast, LandPaths operates the permit-based access program at Willow Creek and conducts guided tours of the Carrington Ranch and Wright Hill Ranch.

Many other organizations contribute to preservation efforts along the Sonoma Coast. These include the California Coastal Conservancy, Wildlife Conservation Board, the National Oceanic and Atmospheric Administration, Coastwalk, and the Gordon and Betty Moore Foundation. In the end, though, preservation depends on the commitment of the public. If you would like to help preserve Sonoma's magnificent coast, consider making a donation or volunteering with any of the groups dedicated to this effort.

Sonoma Coast State Park Hiking Trails

Sonoma Coast offers day hikes for every level of experience, from the wheelchair-accessible path at Vista Trail to the thousand-foot climb of Islands in the Sky Trail. The four primary hiking regions are Bodega Head, Bodega Dunes, the northern coast, and Willow Creek.

At Bodega Head, a loop trail around the point is a great place to enjoy ocean views and watch for coastal birds, seals, sea lions, and whales. Overlook Trail leads north from the parking lot and past the private Bodega Marine Reserve to the little-traveled south end of Bodega Dunes.

Several trails wind through the soft sand at Bodega Dunes, which are broader and higher than they might first seem. Hikers can access the dunes from several locations, while equestrians can access them from the trailhead at Bay Flat Road. If you're looking for solitude, you'll find it here. While you may meet an occasional rider on horseback, you are more likely to see the native deer, rabbits, and foxes than other hikers.

Along the northern coast, the Kortum Trail and Vista Trail take you through windswept, wildflower-covered headlands. The Pomo Canyon and Red Hill Trails climb the coastal hills though open grasslands and redwood forests. You'll find the most strenuous hikes and best ocean views at Willow Creek, where access is limited to holders of permits issued by the non-profit organization LandPaths. This is also the only area in the park suitable for mountain biking.

Trail 1: Bodega Head Loop

Length: 1.8 mile loop (2.0 miles with optional side trip to summit), 1 hour

Difficulty: Easy

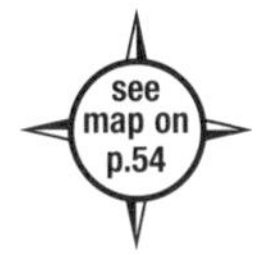

Overview: This relatively level loop circles the southern tip of Bodega Head. It hugs the cliff edges for most of its distance, so keep young children in control. From December through April, you may be lucky enough to glimpse the spouts of California gray whales as they migrate along the coast. At several points along the way, you'll see sheltered beaches 150 feet below you, but the faint volunteer trails down to them aren't maintained by the State and descent is dangerous. Stay on the loop trail–if you really want to frolic in the sand, head for one of the northern beaches.

Directions to Trailhead: Take Highway 1 to the north side of Bodega Bay. Turn west at the large sign labeled BODEGA HEAD–WESTSIDE PARK–MARINAS at Eastshore Road. Follow the road down the hill and turn right at the stop sign. This is Bay Flat Road, which becomes Westshore Road after 0.2 mile. Stay on this road for 3 miles to Campbell Cove, then continue around the hairpin turn sharply right and up the hill. At the Y intersection in the headlands above Campbell Cove, keep right to reach the west parking lot. The trail departs from the southwest corner of the parking lot just past the outhouses.

Trail Description: The trail starts just to the west of the outhouses and heads south along the bluff. At 300 feet, you see a ceremonial tribute to lost fishermen on your left. Continuing southward, at 0.1 mile you see a sandy beach far down the base of the cliff on your right. A rough trail descends part way down the cliff, but it is unsafe to descend. Stay on the bluff and admire this beach from a distance. You may see seals lounging on the sand far below.

At 0.4 mile, a short spur trail branches to a viewpoint on your right. Just beyond, you reach the crest of a slight hill. From here you can first see Bodega Rock rising from the sea to the southeast. Bodega Rock is home to a large colony of seals, and you will often be serenaded by their barks for the next mile of your hike.

The main trail turns east at 0.6 mile, just as another spur trail branches to a viewpoint on the right. Then at 0.7 mile, you may wish to take the side trail on your left to a 204-foot summit. The summit offers spectacular 360-degree views of the Sonoma and Marin coasts and adds

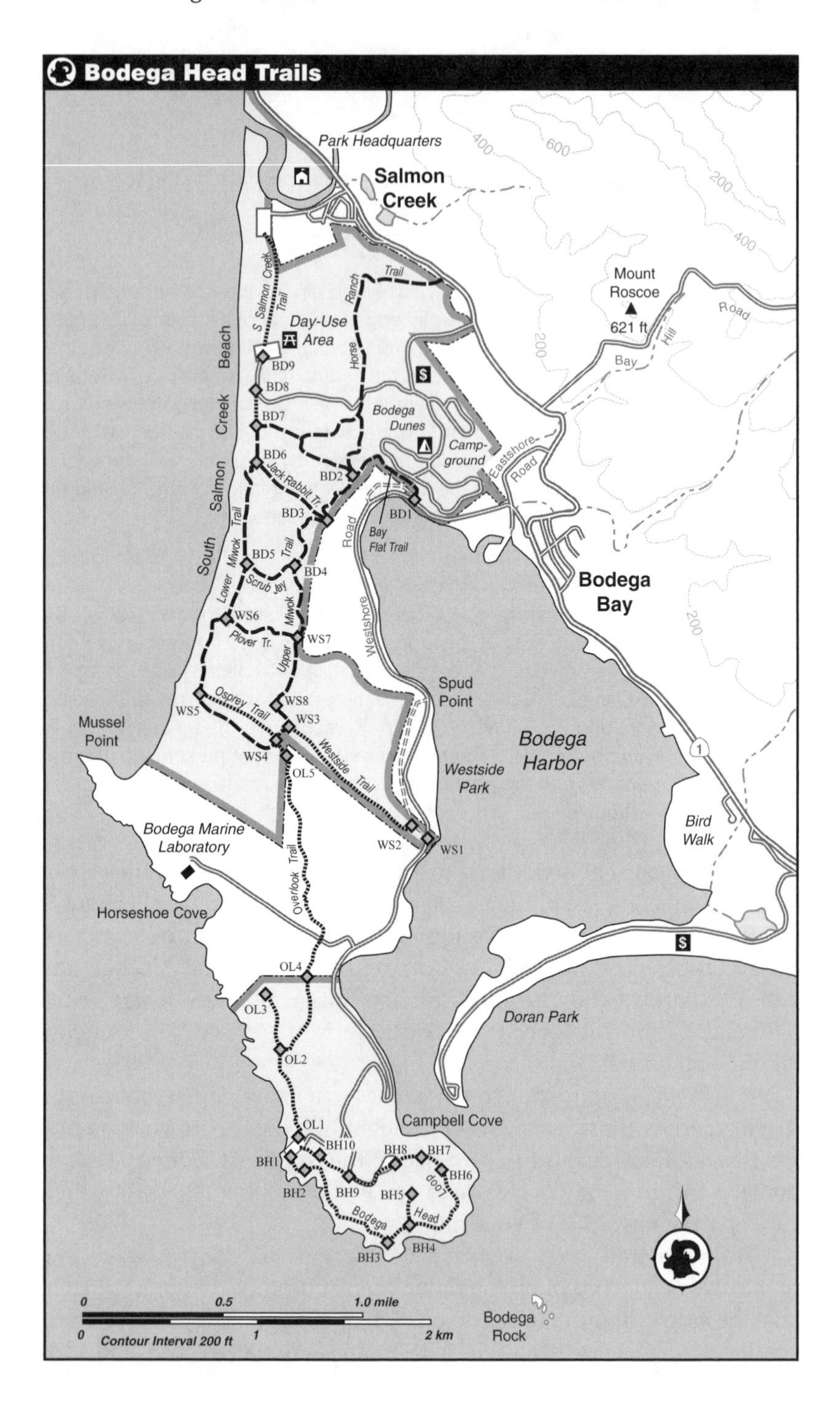
Bodega Head Trails
Park Headquarters
Salmon Creek
Mount Roscoe
621 ft
Bay Hill Road
Day-Use Area
S Salmon Creek Trail
Horse Ranch Trail
South Salmon Creek Beach
Bodega Dunes Campground
Eastshore Road
Jack Rabbit Tr.
Lower Miwok Trail
Upper Miwok Trail
Scrub Jay Trail
Bay Flat Trail
Westshore Road
Plover Tr.
Osprey Trail
Westside Trail
Bodega Bay
Spud Point
Bodega Harbor
Westside Park
Mussel Point
Bodega Marine Laboratory
Overlook Trail
Horseshoe Cove
Bird Walk
Doran Park
Campbell Cove
Bodega Head Loop
Bodega Rock
BD1
BD2
BD3
BD4
BD5
BD6
BD7
BD8
BD9
WS1
WS2
WS3
WS4
WS5
WS6
WS7
WS8
OL1
OL2
OL3
OL4
OL5
BH1
BH2
BH3
BH4
BH5
BH6
BH7
BH8
BH9
BH10
0 0.5 1.0 mile
0 1 2 km
Contour Interval 200 ft

an optional 0.2 mile round trip. In clear weather, Point Reyes Peninsula stretches across the southern horizon, while to the north you can see to Goat Rock and beyond. From the summit, you can return the way you came or continue down the side trail for the shortest path to the east parking lot. The described route returns along the main loop.

At 0.9 mile a marine navigation marker looms directly in front of you, and you begin to see the breakwater of Bodega Harbor. The trail here runs very close to the cliff edge, so be cautious, especially with small children. Continuing across the wildflower-covered headlands, you soon reach an immense cow parsnip forest. In the spring and summer, the white-flowered shoots of these members of the carrot family can climb as high as 10 feet into the air.

You reach the east parking lot at 1.3 miles. Here you'll find excellent views of the harbor and Campbell Cove. You also look down on the fenced-off remains of the infamous Hole-in-the-Head, the only remains of a planned nuclear power plant that was never completed. From this lot, go west along the road to a gated dirt driveway on your left at 1.5 miles. Go around the gate, where you see two trails, a wide dirt road proceeding directly ahead and a narrow trail veering right at a compass bearing of 300°. Take the narrow trail toward an isolated stand of cypress at 1.6 miles. The tangled branches of these trees form a natural fort for children. It's an easy walk from here back to the west lot trailhead.

Trail 1: Bodega Head Loop Waypoints (WGS84 Datum)

Name	Latitude	Longitude	Feature
BH1	N38° 18.202′	W123° 03.875′	Trailhead
BH2	N38° 18.153′	W123° 03.811′	Fisherman's Memorial
BH3	N38° 17.930′	W123° 03.480′	Junction with side trail to viewpoint
BH4	N38° 18.000′	W123° 03.404′	Junction with trail to summit
BH5	N38° 18.085′	W123° 03.392′	Summit
BH6	N38° 18.162′	W123° 03.275′	Picnic table
BH7	N38° 18.201′	W123° 03.350′	Junction with trail towards harbor
BH8	N38° 18.183′	W123° 03.436′	East parking lot and outhouses
BH9	N38° 18.154′	W123° 03.655′	Gated dirt driveway
BH10	N38° 18.187′	W123° 03.771′	Cypress stand with natural fort

Trail 2: Overlook Trail

Length: 3.8 miles round trip from Bodega Head to Bodega Dunes, 2.5 hours. Longer hikes possible by continuing on trails through the dunes.

Difficulty: Moderate

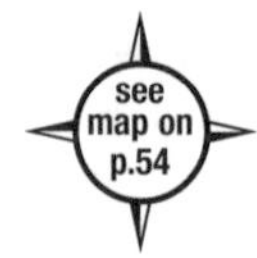

Overview: This trail leads across headlands covered with ice plant, purple seaside daisies, bush lupine, and coastal scrub/grasslands. From December through April, keep an eye open for migrating whales. Part of this trail traverses the Bodega Marine Reserve, a 326-acre laboratory operated by the University of California. The Reserve is otherwise off-limits to the public, so obey the posted signs and stay on the trail along this portion. You can visit the lab when it is open to the public on Fridays from 2 to 4 P.M.; take the marked road west off Westshore Road.

Directions to Trailhead: Same as Trail 1 to the west parking lot. Park at the east end of the lot, away from the ocean. Pick up the trail at the northeast corner of the parking lot.

Trail Description: From the parking lot, follow the path up the bluff. As you climb, you'll have excellent views of the coast on your left and the harbor on your right.

About 0.3 mile from the trailhead, you come to a spur trail on your left. Take this path to an overlook with a good view of Horseshoe Cove and the Marine Reserve Laboratory at 0.6 mile; the marine lab staff asks that you not proceed past the overlook.

Returning to the main trail, turn left to begin a steady descent, reaching the Marine Lab boundary at 1.1 miles. Stay on the trail while you traverse this property. As you hike, notice how the terrain changes from coastal scrub to grass-covered dunes. Follow the trail markers to reach the southern end of Bodega Dunes beach, exiting Marine Lab property at 1.9 miles. From here, you can either return the way you came or continue along the dunes trails for a longer hike. Refer to Trail 4, Bodega Dunes Loop via Westside Trail, for a description of the hike beyond its junction with Overlook Trail.

Trail 2: Overlook Trail Waypoints (WGS84 Datum)

Name	Latitude	Longitude	Feature
OL1	N38° 18.242′	W123° 03.851′	Trailhead
OL2	N38° 18.515′	W123° 03.913′	Junction with spur trail to overlook
OL3	N38° 18.686′	W123° 03.969′	Bodega Marine Laboratory overlook
OL4	N38° 18.747′	W123° 03.803′	Entry into Bodega Marine Laboratory property
OL5	N38° 19.381′	W123° 03.882′	Exit from Bodega Marine Laboratory property

Trail 3: Miwok Loop Trail via Bay Flat Trailhead

Length: 3.2 miles to Day Use Picnic Area, 2 hours. Additional 1.3 miles to return to start, 1 hour. Shorter hikes also possible.

Difficulty: Strenuous (due to walking on soft sand)

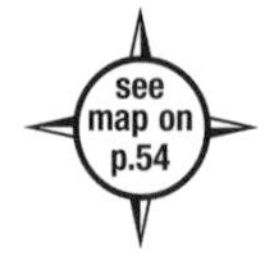

Overview: Hikers may be tempted to avoid this trail because it is a main horse path to the dunes, but don't be discouraged. On a sunny Saturday in June, I didn't encounter another person, either on horseback or on foot, during my entire hike. I frequently use this trail for field training students in my GPS navigation classes. If there aren't a lot of horse trailers parked in the lot, you should be safe enough.

This is a great way to see the less-traveled areas of Bodega Dunes. You will walk through a vast tract of shrub-covered dunes, with many spectacular views of the Sonoma Coast. After an initial 100-foot climb the elevation changes are gradual, but hiking through the soft sand can be strenuous, making this a much more exhausting hike than you may think. Take plenty of water and snacks, and plan to spend at least 4 hours to cover the entire distance, including time for a picnic lunch.

Although the described hike is 4.5 miles long, you have several opportunities for a shorter hike. There are also numerous other ways to enter this trail, including South Salmon Creek Trail out of the Bodega Dunes day-use area, Westside Trail from West Shore Road, and Overlook Trail from Bodega Head.

Directions to Trailhead: Follow the directions to Bodega Head on Page 53, but rather than driving all the way to the Head, park at the large dirt parking area 0.2 mile beyond the stop sign at the bottom of the hill as you turn onto Bay Flat Road. This is Bay Flat Trailhead, the main equestrian access to Bodega Dunes, and you may see horse trailers in this lot. There is no fee to enter the dunes from here.

Trail Description: The route starts at the north end of the horse-trailer parking lot, just beyond a dirt road. Go through the opening in the fence and turn sharply left. The level ground quickly turns to deep sand visibly churned by horses' hooves. Keeping left, you see the campground on your right and private property across the fence to your left. At 0.3 mile you reach the base of a large dune. Although athletic people may be tempted to climb the steep face of this dune, the actual trail turns left, quickly climbing 100 feet up the back of the dunes. Continue through rolling dunes covered with grass and yellow bush lupine until reaching the junction with Upper Miwok Trail at 0.4 mile.

Keep left and head in a southerly direction. At 0.6 mile, you come to the junction with Jack Rabbit Trail on your right. This is your first chance for a shorter hike—Jack Rabbit Trail is a shortcut to Lower Miwok Trail.

This hike continues south along Upper Miwok Trail, where you quickly reach a side trail continuing directly ahead. The main trail, though, makes a sharp right turn and begins climbing. Stay on the main trail, as the side trail soon becomes faint and disappears. You soon turn sharply left and traverse a deep sand gulley through the dunes. Be alert for horses in this stretch and stand quietly to the side if necessary to let them pass.

Emerging from the gulley, you come to a broad, sandy plain. Notice the dense vegetation, including native yellow bush lupine and ice plant as well as various introduced grasses that help stabilize the shifting dunes. Listen for sounds of the surf far down to your right. At 0.9 mile you reach the junction with Scrub Jay Trail. This is your next chance for a shorter hike.

This hike continues south. At 1.2 miles you reach the junction with Plover Trail, a third opportunity for a shorter hike. Continuing straight ahead, you reach the intersection with Westside Trail at 1.5 miles and the junction with Osprey Trail and Overlook Trail at 1.6 miles. The described hike turns right along Osprey Trail toward the ocean. This lightly traveled section of the dunes is a good place to look for some of its more reclusive inhabitants, including jackrabbits, badgers, raccoons, and foxes.

At 1.9 miles you reach the junction with Lower Miwok Trail. Turn right and begin your return journey. Follow Lower Miwok Trail north to Plover Trail at 2.2 miles and Scrub Jay Trail at 2.4 miles. Continuing north, the trail remains fairly straight and level until you reach a broad dune running perpendicular to your path. Here the trail winds through a stand of cypress trees and emerges at the junction with Jack Rabbit Trail at 2.8 miles and the junction with Horse Ranch Trail at 2.9 miles.

As you continue north along the broad trail, notice the numerous shell fragments in the sand at 3.0 miles. Just to your left is a mound of dark soil and shells. This is a Native American midden, or refuse heap, that survives from when this region was the domain of the Coast Miwoks. Middens are protected by law, so admire, but do not disturb, this archaeologically significant site.

You reach the paved road at 3.1 miles. Follow the road to the day-use picnic area at 3.2 miles where you will find wooden tables, fire rings, elevated barbecues, and outhouses. Take time to rest and enjoy a picnic lunch here, then explore the wooden boardwalk to the beach.

When you are ready to leave, return along the paved road to the Lower Miwok trail junction on your right at 0.1 mile. From there, take the trail through the sand to the junction with Jack Rabbit Trail at 0.4 mile. Turn left and follow Jack Rabbit Trail back to Upper Miwok Trail at 0.7 mile. Turn left onto Upper Miwok Trail to the junction with Bay Flat Trail at 0.9 mile, then along Bay Flat Trail back to the parking lot at 1.3 miles, for a total hike of 4.5 miles.

Trail 3: Miwok Loop Trail via Bay Flat Trail Waypoints (WGS84 Datum)

Name	Latitude	Longitude	Feature
BD1	N38° 20.150′	W123° 03.361′	Bay Flat Road Trailhead
BD2	N38° 20.240′	W123° 03.620′	Junction of Bay Flat and Upper Miwok Trails
BD3	N38° 20.108′	W123° 03.731′	Junction of Upper Miwok and Jack Rabbit Trails
BD4	N38° 19.957′	W123° 03.859′	Junction of Upper Miwok and Scrub Jay Trails
BD5	N38° 19.976′	W123° 04.051′	Junction of Lower Miwok and Scrub Jay Trails
BD6	N38° 20.273′	W123° 04.011′	Junction of Lower Miwok and Jack Rabbit Trails
BD7	N38° 20.388′	W123° 04.008′	Junction of Lower Miwok and Horse Ranch Trails
BD8	N38° 20.497′	W123° 04.011′	Junction of Lower Miwok Trail with road
BD9	N38° 20.618′	W123° 03.997′	Day Use Area

Trail 4: Bodega Dunes Loop via Westside Trail

Length: 2.7 miles, 1.5 hours. Longer hikes possible by continuing through the dunes.

Difficulty: Strenuous (due to walking on soft sand)

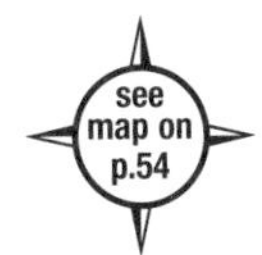

Overview: This little-used trail lets you explore some of the more remote areas of Bodega Dunes. Although you never climb more than 100 feet, your entire route is on soft sand, making it a fairly strenuous hike. Westside Trail itself is simply an access route to the dunes. It connects to Upper Miwok Trail after a half mile. This hike follows Westside Trail to its end and continues on Miwok Trail over the southern portion of the Miwok Loop Trail described in Trail 3. It then makes a loop and returns back along Westside Trail. However, if you are feeling particularly energetic you can extend your hike farther along Lower Miwok Trail to as far as the Day Use Area, with several other opportunities for an earlier return.

Directions to Trailhead: Follow the directions to Bodega Head on Page 53, but rather than driving all the way to the Head, drive 1.8 miles beyond the stop sign at Bay Flat Road. Just after you pass Westside Park, look for a dirt road on your right, where a lone cypress tree stands in front of a sandy berm. Turn here and park near the cypress tree.

Trail Description: The trailhead lies next to the cypress tree. In the dry season, walk to the right of the tree, across a seasonal wetland dominated by Pacific silverweed, then up the side of the sand berm. In the wet season, you will have to walk to the left of the cypress and make your way carefully through reeds to the top of the berm.

Once on top, your trail climbs steadily as it heads northwest toward the main body of the dunes. Initially, ice plant and coast buckwheat line the trail. At 0.4 mile, you enter dense stands of dune grass. These imported grasses were planted in the middle of the 20th century to help stabilize the dunes and prevent them from silting up Bodega Harbor.

Westside Trail ends at the junction with Upper Miwok Trail at 0.6 mile. Turn left here. You quickly come to a second trail junction with trails going in three directions. Overlook Trail to Bodega Head (Trail 2) is on the left. Miwok Loop Riding/Hiking Trail continues straight ahead, and Osprey Trail is on the right. You are more likely to encounter equestrians than hikers in this part of the dunes, so turn right and follow Osprey Trail (horses not permitted) west toward the beach. As you descend through bush lupine and dune grass, you have a grand view of the coast from Bodega Head on the south to Goat Rock far to the north. This stretch of dunes is a good place to look for some of its more reclusive inhabitants, including foxes, raccoons, and badgers.

You reach another three-way junction at 1.0 mile, indicated by a series of low wooden railings. Two picnic tables with hitching rails lie directly ahead, beside a short spur trail to Salmon Creek Beach. Lower Miwok Trail enters on the left, crosses the junction, and continues north. Turn right here and follow Lower Miwok Trail to its junction with Plover Trail at 1.4 miles. Although you are welcome to continue on Lower Miwok Trail, this hike turns right and heads east up Plover Trail to the top of the dunes.

After climbing 100 feet, you reach the junction with Upper Miwok Trail at 1.7 miles. Turn right here to continue your loop. Just before 2.0 miles, a broad trail on the left goes down the side of a dune and disappears. Keep left on the main trail, where you again reach the junction with Westside Trail at 2.1 miles. Turn left here and return down the berm to reach the trailhead at 2.7 miles.

Trail 4: Bodega Dunes Loop via Westside Trail Waypoints (WGS84 Datum)

Name	Latitude	Longitude	Feature
WS1	N38° 19.144′	W123° 03.335′	Turnoff from West Shore Road to Westside Trailhead
WS2	N38° 19.183′	W123° 03.380′	Westside Trail trailhead and parking area
WS3	N38° 19.486′	W123° 03.884′	Junction of Westside and Upper Miwok Trails
WS4	N38° 19.444′	W123° 03.938′	Junction of Osprey and Upper Miwok Trails
WS5	N38° 19.564′	W123° 04.237′	Junction of Osprey and Lower Miwok Trails
WS6	N38° 19.816′	W123° 04.134′	Junction of Plover and Lower Miwok Trails
WS7	N38°19.754′	W123° 03.850′	Junction of Plover and Upper Miwok Trails
WS8	N38° 19.559′	W123° 03.949′	Trail junction – keep left

Trail 5: Kortum Trail: Shell Beach north to Blind Beach

Length: 4.6 miles round trip to Blind Beach, 2 hours. Deduct 0.6 mile and 200 feet elevation change if you stop at the Blind Beach parking lot and return from there.

Difficulty: Moderate (steep from Blind Beach parking lot to Blind Beach)

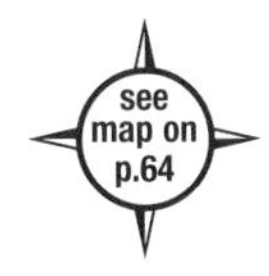

Overview: This pleasant trail from Shell Beach to Blind Beach extends along the coastal bluffs with excellent views of the rugged coastline. You will also pass the probable site of Pleistocene "rubbing rocks" frequented by prehistoric mammoths. You will have little shelter from the blowing winds, so save this hike for calm weather. The trail is named for former Sonoma County Supervisor Bill Kortum. In the early 1970s he helped lead the effort to stop construction of housing developments that would have destroyed the natural beauty of this coast.

Directions to Trailhead: From Bodega Bay, drive 7 miles north on Highway 1 to the Shell Beach parking lot just west of the highway at milepost marker 18.22. The Kortum Trail crosses at the west edge of the lot. Look for the sign just north of the outhouses.

Trail Description: From the northwest side of the Shell Beach parking lot, follow a well-maintained gravel/dirt trail north through open grassland and coyote brush. At 0.1 mile you reach a fence line where the trail splits three ways. A wooden signpost labeled OVERLOOK points to a trail on your left that heads directly west toward the bluffs. A short walk of a few hundred feet along this trail ends at a point overlooking numerous sea stacks, where on a clear day you can see Bodega Head to the south.

A second trail heads northwest across the headlands, while a broad third trail leads directly north for the shortest path to Blind Beach. Unless you are in a hurry, take the second trail northwest toward the bluffs. In spring and summer, you will see a multitude of flowers including cow parsnip, twinberry, and purple thistle. As the trail curves around a gully at 0.3 mile, stay to the left and follow the coastline.

At 0.4 mile you rejoin the broad third trail and head northeast toward the flank of Red Hill, looming in the distance across Highway 1. A boardwalk at 0.5 mile extends over wetlands and a seasonal creek with dune grass, thistle, and blackberries. The boardwalk crosses

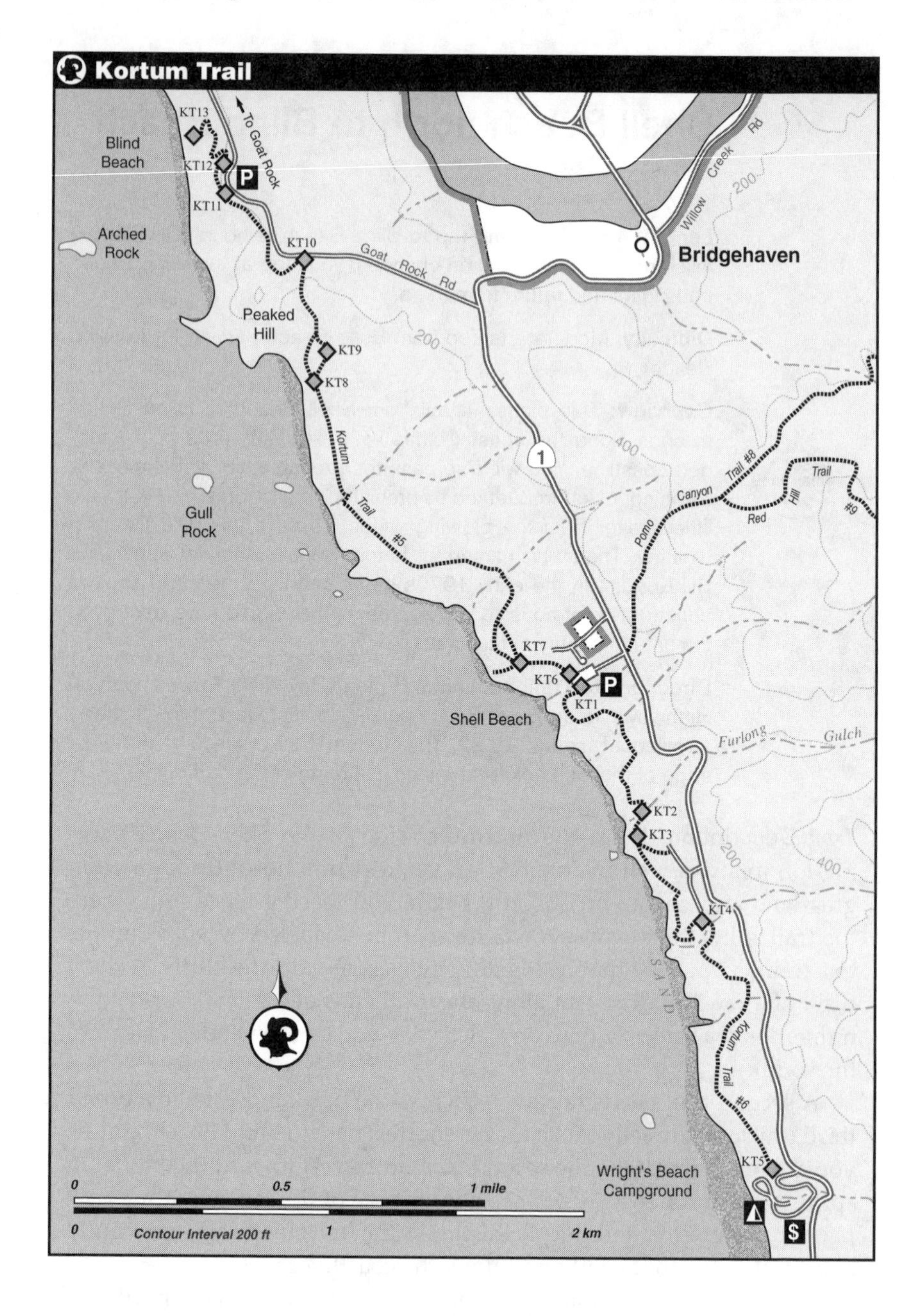
Kortum Trail
KT13
To Goat Rock
Blind Beach
KT12
P
KT11
Arched Rock
KT10
Goat Rock Rd
Willow Creek Rd
200
Bridgehaven
Peaked Hill
200
KT9
KT8
Kortum Trail #5
1
400
Trail #8
Canyon
Pomo
Red Hill Trail #9
Gull Rock
KT7
KT6
P
KT1
Shell Beach
Furlong Gulch
KT2
KT3
200
400
KT4
SAND
Kortum Trail #6
KT5
Wright's Beach Campground
$
0
0.5
1 mile
0
Contour Interval 200 ft
1
2 km

another seasonal creek just before it ends at 0.6 mile. Here, the trail turns due west. When I hiked this trail in late fall, I counted three harmless garter snakes sunning themselves along this stretch of the path.

You reach another 500-foot long boardwalk at 0.8 mile, stretching through dune grass and blackberry vines. These boardwalks were installed to protect seasonal wetlands, so stay on the trail along this stretch. As the boardwalk ends, your trail turns northward. The white, guano-covered surface of Arched Rock lies offshore directly ahead.

You descend a gully and cross a wooden bridge at 1.0 mile, with Gull Rock to your left. Flora along this stretch includes purple seaside daisies, cow parsnip, leather ferns, and vetch. A large on-shore sea stack lies ahead on your right, accessed by a side trail at 1.1 miles. Adventurous souls have been known to scramble to its top for great views of the coastline, but this is a dangerous proposition. Another smaller sea stack, split down the middle, is visible ahead. A side trail at 1.3 miles branches off to this split rock. Take this trail, which passes directly through the middle of the split at 1.4 miles.

These rocks, known as Sunset Rocks, are popular spots for rock climbers. A hundred thousand years ago, all but their tops were under water. In the interim, the relentless movement of the San Andreas Fault has pushed the land upward to its present level. Recently, a theory has been proposed that Sunset Rocks were "rubbing rocks" frequented by Pleistocene mammoths (see sidebar on page 66).

After passing through the split rocks, head northwest and rejoin the main trail at 1.5 miles. You begin a steady ascent up the side of Peaked Hill, passing fenced-off areas to your left that are study sites for raptor research. As you approach Goat Rock Road, you have good views south to Bodega Head and, on a clear day, all the way to Point Reyes 30 miles away.

You reach the top of the climb at 1.8 miles, passing through a saddle between Peaked Hill on your left and a smaller, unnamed peak on your right. A side trail branches off to the top of Peaked Hill.

Continuing on, you descend through coyote brush toward Blind Beach. The trail reaches Goat Rock Road at 2 miles and the Blind Beach parking lot soon after. In early 2008, this parking lot was the site of tragic late-night violence when members of an Asian street gang shot and killed a former member who was scheduled to testify against them. A park ranger who happened along the scene minutes later radioed a description of the escaping vehicle, and the occupants were quickly captured.

Rubbing Rocks—A Prehistoric Landmark

The towering blueschist pillars known as Sunset Rocks have long been popular with rock climbers. Recent evidence now suggests these ancient sea stacks might well have been popular long before the first climbers scrambled to their tops. Breck Parkman, Senior State Archaeologist for California State Parks, believes these were once "rubbing rocks" frequented by large Ice Age mammals including mammoths, mastodons, bison, and ground sloths.

Parkman points to large areas of the rock surface that have been polished smooth up to a height of 14 feet above ground. Microscopic examination of these surfaces shows patterns of scratches similar to those made by modern elephants rubbing on scratching posts. Such scratches, caused by small particles of grit that get embedded in the animals' fur after wallowing, have characteristic patterns not consistent with natural weathering. While it is possible domestic cattle that previously grazed here could have polished the lower surfaces, they can't account for those polished surfaces 14 feet high. Since Parkman first proposed his theory in 2001, a stream of experts have examined the rocks and generally come away believers.

At the close of the last Ice Age 10,000 years ago, sea levels were much lower than today. The Sonoma Coast was part of a broad, grassy savannah that stretched as far out as the Farallon Islands. Sunset Rocks sit along a likely game trail through a pass in the nearby hills. The rocks would have been a natural attraction for the giant animals. Parkman points to a nearby depression, an isolated wetland of uncertain origin, as the possible location of an ancient wallow. Although no mammoth bones have yet been found in the immediate area, they have been recovered elsewhere along the coast.

Parkman has done a number of surveys of the site, including an inconclusive small-scale chemical analysis. He has led several excavations that have unearthed a large number of Paleolithic arrowheads and stone tools, but as of yet, no mammoth bones. As Parkman says, "instead of finding paleontological evidence of the megafauna, I got buried (no pun intended) beneath a lot of archaeological evidence." Once he has completed the archaeological analysis, he will return looking for bones.

The biggest threat to the rocks today is damage by careless climbers and souvenir hunters. In the years since the theory was first publicized, the number of chips from rockhounds' hammers has continued to grow. If you go, remember this is an irreplaceable part of prehistory, so look, but don't damage the rocks.

If you want to descend all the way to Blind Beach, take the trail at the northeast side of the lot just beside the dual outhouse. This trail winds 200 feet down to the beach. "Floating" wooden stairs ease the last 20 feet of this descent. At this point you have traversed a total distance of 2.3 miles. Unless you have arranged a car shuttle at the Blind Beach parking lot, you will now need to retrace your path back to Shell Beach.

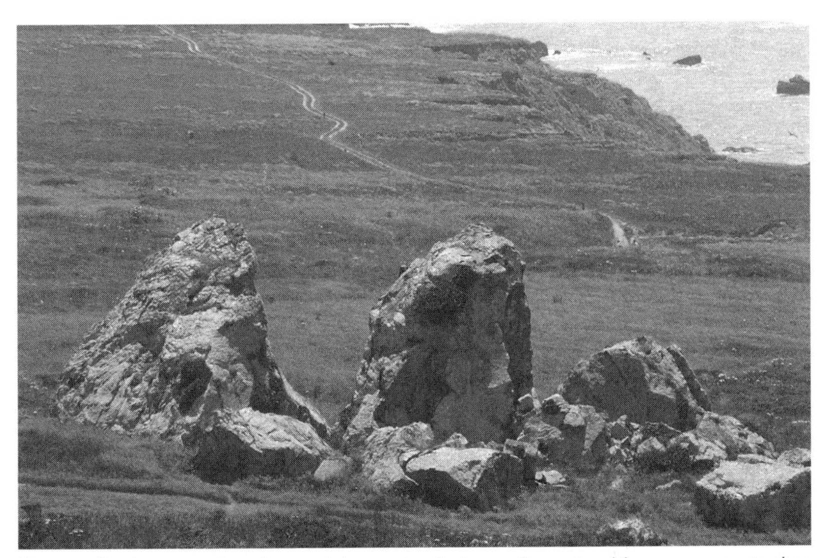

Sunset Rocks are a favorite spot for rock climbers. Recent evidence suggests they may also have served as rubbing rocks for ice-age mammoths. Kortum Trail can be seen in the background.

Trails 5–6: **Kortum Trail Waypoints (WGS84 Datum)**

Name	Latitude	Longitude	Feature
KT1	N38° 25.076′	W123° 06.267′	South Trailhead at Shell Beach
KT2	N38° 24.814′	W123° 06.077′	Junction with side trail to Furlong Gulch beach.
KT3	N38° 24.763′	W123° 06.075′	Trail junction. Keep right to stay along bluffs.
KT4	N38° 24.587′	W123° 05.910′	Junction with main trail at south end of Carlevaro Way.
KT5	N38° 24.086′	W123° 05.720′	Trailhead above Wright's Beach.
KT6	N38° 25.088′	W123° 06.278′	North Trailhead at Shell Beach.
KT7	N38° 25.117′	W123° 06.406′	Three-way trail junction. Kortum Trail is middle fork.
KT8	N38° 25.693′	W123° 06.966′	Junction with side trail to Sunset Rocks.
KT9	N38° 25.760′	W123° 06.935′	Sunset Rocks.
KT10	N38° 25.937′	W123° 07.023′	Junction with side trail to road.
KT11	N38° 26.076′	W123° 07.210′	Trailhead at Goat Rock Road
KT12	N38° 26.139′	W123° 07.220′	Trailhead from parking area to Blind Beach.
KT13	N38° 26.193′	W123° 07.294′	Trailhead at Blind Beach

Trail 6: Kortum Trail: Shell Beach south to Wright's Beach

Length: 4.4 miles round trip, 2 hours

Difficulty: Moderate

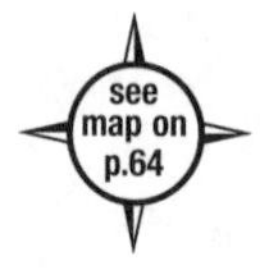

Overview: In spring and summer, the coastal headlands along this reasonably easy trail from Shell Beach to Wright's Beach are blanketed with a spectacular explosion of wildflowers. Some of the numerous types you'll see include Douglas iris, buttercup, sticky monkeyflower, cow parsnip, flowering currant, purple bush lupine, Indian paintbrush, salmonberry, purple seaside daisy, coast buckwheat, and sea thrift. For a longer hike, you can combine this hike with Trail 5. To cover the entire route, start at either the Blind Beach parking lot and hike south or the Wright's Beach parking lot and hike north.

Directions to Trailhead: Same as Trail 5. The trail departs from the southwest end of the parking lot near the outhouses.

Trail Description. From the trailhead at the southwest edge of the parking lot, descend down a gulch along a single-track dirt trail. Cross a wooden bridge and go up the side of the gulch. As you ascend, you have a nice view of Shell Beach on the right and Peaked Hill farther north. At 0.2 mile the trail curves left, heading straight for the highway and Red Hill beyond. You quickly reach a broad trail heading directly south, but stay on the narrow trail east and enter a forest of chest-high coyote brush.

The trail eventually curves southeast. At 0.3 mile you make a steep descent into an unnamed gulley and cross a wooden footbridge. As you climb out the other side, you have good views of the ocean below. You cross an old road and then curve right, heading due south. As you reach the edge of the bluff, you curve left to follow the bluffs. The trail here can be soggy after recent rains.

At 0.5 mile you begin a long descent into Furlong Gulch, passing cow parsnip, bush lupine, and coyote brush as you wind down the side of the gulch. Cross a long wooden footbridge across the gulch, then a second shorter bridge. Immediately after the second bridge, a trail on your right heads over to the beach, which is well worth a short side trip.

Follow the trail up the south side of the gulch. At the top, a wide trail on your left leads to Carlevaro Way, a remnant from an aborted housing development. While you can take that trail for the shortest path, the described route stays to the right, following the edge of the bluffs. Wild radish blooms profusely along this stretch of the trail.

At 0.8 mile, you pass a sea stack in the making. Storm seas are eroding the softer sediments surrounding a rocky point. Perhaps in a thousand years this point will be a true sea stack surrounded by the ocean.

The trail now curves east around a willow thicket. You get your first glimpse of the ice plant (also known as sea fig), a species imported from South Africa to help stabilize sand dunes across the State. Today, sea fig is considered an unwelcome invasive species that displaces native plants.

An ancient wooden post at 0.9 mile marks the trail as it curves left, where you have a great view of the long, isolated extension of Wrights Beach. From here, you can see from Fort Ross on the north all the way to Point Reyes far to the south. At 1.0 mile, you reach a ravine. Although a faint trail leads down into it, it is impassible for much of the year, so turn sharply left and head north, then east through willows, coyote brush, and beach strawberry. You reach the broad trail at 1.1 miles at the south end of Carlevaro Way. To your left are two houses that now serve as residences for state park personnel. Turn right and follow the main trail south.

You reach a well-maintained side trail to the beach at 1.3 miles and pass beside a large eucalyptus tree at 1.4 miles, just before coming to a 500-foot-long boardwalk over seasonal wetlands. Cross under an old telephone line at 1.6 miles and look for patches of yarrow, with its distinctive white flowers and lacy leaves, along the trail. Follow the trail, now an old dirt road, all the way to a wooden gate at Wright's Beach Road at 1.9 miles. From here, continue on down the road to reach Wright's Beach at 2.2 miles, where you can enjoy a picnic and explore the sand before returning the way you came.

Trail 7: Vista Trail

Length: 0.8 mile, 30 minutes

Difficulty: Easy

Overview: This paved loop trail is accessible to the disabled. The trail has great views of the coast and is a good place to watch for hawks. The entire trail extends across grassland and is reasonably level throughout, with picnic tables at several spots along the way. This is an ideal trail for families with small children.

Directions to Trailhead: From Jenner, drive 4 miles north on Highway 1 to the signed turnoff on your left near milepost 25.52. A good parking lot with a dozen spaces and a dual outhouse is located well off the highway.

Trail Description: The trailhead is at the south side of the parking lot. Take the fractured asphalt path southeast through the grassland. Some of the wildflowers you may see here include yarrow, California poppy, suncups, blue-eyed grass, and Douglas iris. At 0.1 mile you reach a trail junction. Keep right, heading west past coyote brush and native grasses. Your trail quickly curves left and passes a picnic bench with a great view of the ocean and surrounding countryside. Goat Rock and Bodega Head are visible to the south, while to the east, you see several homes built on secluded settings in the hills.

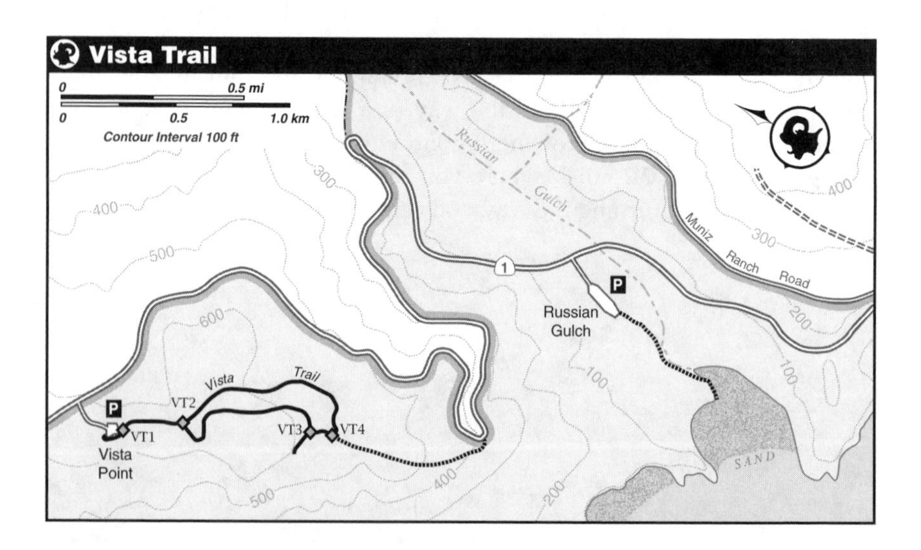

At 0.3 mile, your trail curves back right to pass on the east side of a bluff. You quickly reach another trail junction. Take this spur trail west to a wooden observation deck and a disabled-accessible bench where you have excellent ocean views.

Return to the main loop at 0.4 mile and continue south to another picnic table just beyond. Just as the main trail curves east, a narrow dirt trail heads south toward the cliff. If you choose to take this optional 0.4-mile side trip, you will quickly make a strenuous 200-foot descent to a parking area beside a hairpin curve on Highway 1.

The main trail curves east and then north through the grassland. You reach another picnic table at 0.6 mile, return back to the first trail junction at 0.7 mile, and end your hike at the trailhead at 0.8 mile.

Trail 7: Vista Trail Waypoints (WGS84 Datum)

Name	Latitude	Longitude	Feature
VT1	N38° 28.661′ N	W123° 09.762′	Vista Trail trailhead
VT2	N38° 28.599′ N	W123° 09.717′	Junction with Vista Trail loop. Keep right.
VT3	N38° 28.456′ N	W123° 09.645′	Junction with side trail to scenic overlook
VT4	N38° 28.430′ N	W123° 09.630′	Junction with rough side trail down to Highway 1

Trail 8: Dr. David Joseph Memorial Pomo Canyon Trail

Length: 6 miles round trip from Pomo Canyon Campground to Shell Beach and back, 3.5 hours

Difficulty: Strenuous

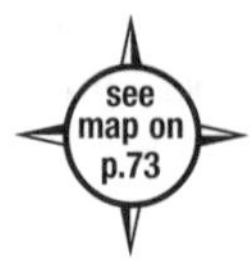

Overview: This quiet trail, a former Native American trading route, climbs 700 feet through redwood forests and grassy hillsides before descending to Highway 1 across from Shell Beach. Named after an early environmentalist, it gives you excellent views of the coast from several locations along the way. This description covers the trail starting from the Pomo Canyon Campground. Trail 9 is a variant that starts from Shell Beach and loops via Red Hill.

Directions to Trailhead: Follow the directions to the Pomo Canyon Environmental Camp on Page 50. The trail begins at the west end of the parking lot, where you must self-register and pay the day-use fee. When the campground is closed in winter, you'll have to park at the gate and walk the level half-mile dirt road to the trailhead.

Trail Description: The trail begins at the west end of the parking lot, passing outhouses on your left as you enter the environmental camp. Campsites lie on either side of the trail here. Notice the growth patterns of the redwoods in this grove. Many of the trees are growing in circular patterns around a central core. These are fairy rings, which occur when a fallen tree regenerates from sprouts around the periphery of its stump. Redwoods are one of the few conifers that can develop from sprouts as well as seeds. These growth patterns confirm that this area was once logged; you can still see occasional stumps along the trail.

Continue a steady climb through the shaded forest. Watch for poison oak along the trailside. At 0.6 mile you reach the junction with Red Hill Trail (Trail 9) on your left. Although you are welcome to take that route to a view at the top of Red Hill, this hike continues straight ahead.

Eventually the ascent eases as you break out of the forest. The trail levels out at about 0.8 mile. On your right is a rock outcrop with a short volunteer trail to its top. With its panoramic view out to Jenner and the northern coast, this is a good spot to stop for lunch or a snack. Continuing along the main trail, you pass through several stands of fir and bay laurel, then emerge into a region of rolling grasslands. In the spring and summer, impressive wildflower displays can be seen here.

On your left is an old fence line, now nearly obscured by poison oak. At several points along the way you cross small wooden bridges over babbling brooks. On your right, you'll have excellent views of Jenner and the mouth of the Russian River.

Finally, after hiking just over 2 miles, you reach the top of the ridgeline. On a clear day, you are treated to a spectacular view of the southern coast all the way to Point Reyes. Notice the eroded rock outcroppings on your left, ancient sea stacks that have been lifted 600 feet by the relentless motion of the San Andreas Fault. Directly below, you have a good view of the offshore sea stack known as Gull Rock.

If you don't have a car waiting for you at Shell Beach, this might be a good place to turn back. The trail from here quickly descends to the sea through open grassland, so the last mile of the hike will add a 500-foot climb to your return trek.

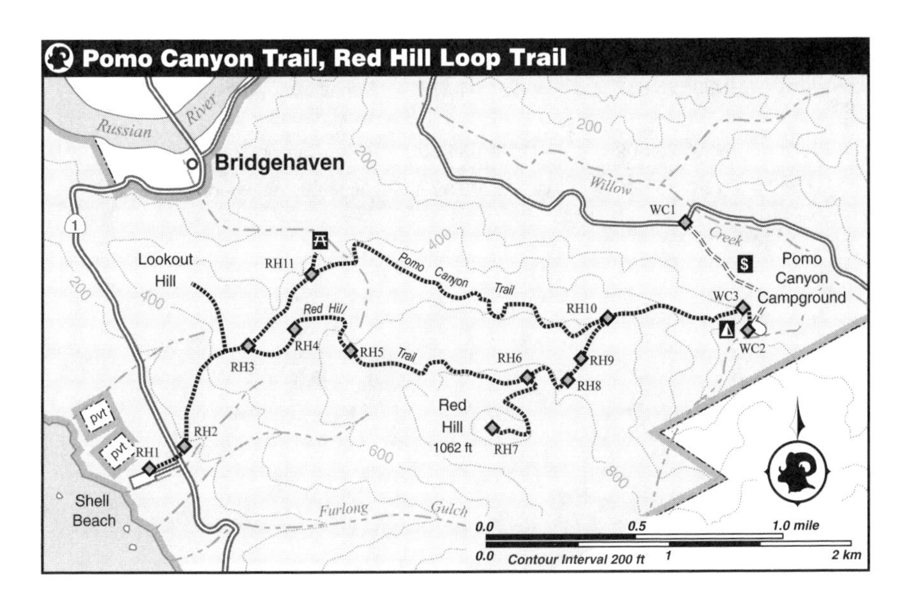

Trails 8–9: Pomo Canyon-Red Hill Loop Waypoints (WGS84 Datum)

Name	Latitude	Longitude	Feature
RH1	N38° 25.095′	W123° 06.239′	Shell Beach parking lot
RH2	N38° 25.143′	W123° 06.107′	Pomo Canyon Trailhead
RH3	N38° 25.460′	W123° 05.856′	Junction with Red Hill Trail
RH4	N38° 25.501′	W123° 05.678′	Outstanding view of Jenner and Russian River
RH5	N38° 25.444′	W123° 05.462′	Hiker's gate through wire fence
RH6	N38° 25.357′	W123° 04.801′	Junction with side trail to top of Red Hill
RH7	N38° 25.223′	W123° 04.928′	Top of Red Hill
RH8	N38° 25.338′	W123° 04.682′	Wooden foot bridge across gully
RH9	N38° 25.386′	W123° 04.618′	Hiker's gate through wooden fence
RH10	N38° 25.531′	W123° 04.489′	Junction with Pomo Canyon Trail
RH11	N38° 25.666′	W123° 05.613′	Trail to picnic table on nearby knoll
WC1	N38° 25.807′	W123° 04.213′	Turnoff from Willow Creek Road to campground
WC2	N38° 25.509′	W123° 03.950′	Pomo Canyon Trailhead
WC3	N38° 25.566′	W123° 03.977′	Numerous redwood fairy rings

Trail 9: Red Hill Loop Trail

Length: 5.5 miles round trip including side loop to top of Red Hill, 3 hours

Difficulty: Strenuous

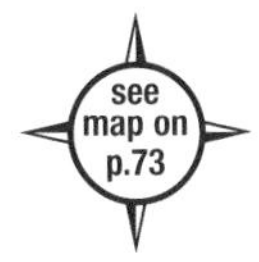

Overview: In 2000, the State acquired the 910-acre Sequeira Ranch, which includes 1062-ft Red Hill. The 2.3-mile hike to the peak through open grassland and occasional forest leads to magnificent views of the coast from Point Reyes to Fort Ross. Follow Pomo Canyon Trail for the first half mile, then take Red Hill Trail to the peak. Complete the loop by continuing along Red Hill Trail until it rejoins Pomo Canyon Trail, which leads you back to Shell Beach. Although this trail starts from Shell Beach, you can also reach the peak from the Pomo Canyon Environmental Camp as described in Trail 8.

Directions to Trailhead: Drive to the Shell Beach parking lot as described in Trail 5. Park at the east end of the parking lot and walk back to the highway. Carefully cross the road and walk to the metal gate at the trailhead. Distances for this hike are measured from the parking lot, not the trailhead.

Trail Description: The trailhead lies 0.1 mile east of the parking lot, directly across Highway 1. Be careful to watch for cars as you cross the highway. Enter beside the gate and pass a sign warning of mountain lions. (Although you would be exceedingly lucky to see one, it is best to observe the cautions listed on the sign.) The trail climbs northeast, then east up an old dirt road with occasional remnants of asphalt. The open grass hillside is dotted with bracken ferns, purple thistle, birdsfoot lotus, and coyote brush. Looking back toward the ocean you have great views of the Pacific with Bodega Head to the south and Gull Rock and Sonoma's Lost Coast to the north.

You pass under a power line at 0.4 mile and reach the top of the initial climb at 0.5 mile. A side trail to Lookout Hill at 0.6 mile takes off to the left, while a prehistoric sea stack, now lifted several hundred feet above sea level, looms directly ahead. You quickly come to the junction with Red Hill Trail, marked by a wooden post. Follow Red Hill Trail as it curves south, then east along a broad dirt road. You begin a gradual climb between the sea stacks, with yellow monkeyflower, wild carrot, and poison oak visible along the slopes of the southern stack.

At 0.8 mile you have an excellent view of Jenner and the Russian River on the north. Directly below lies Pomo Canyon Trail, which will be your return route. Continuing the climb, you enter a cow parsnip forest with spectacular white blooms in spring and early summer. The trail turns south at 1.1 miles through coyote brush and occasional poison oak. As it turns back east, Red Hill looms directly ahead, distinguished by a dense stand of redwoods on its northeastern flank. You will pass through the edge of this forest shortly.

You reach a fence line at 1.2 miles, where a hiker's gate allows you to pass. As you continue climbing through barren grasslands, you enjoy grand views of the hills north of the Russian River.

You briefly enter the edge of the redwood forest at 1.6 miles, continuing a slow, steady climb. At 1.9 miles, you reach the junction with a side trail on your right to the top of Red Hill. Take this trail, which again curves briefly through the edge of the forest. As you emerge, you can see distant Mt. St. Helena to your left beyond a nearby range of hills.

You reach the windswept top of Red Hill at 2.3 miles. From here, on a clear day you have spectacular views of the coast all the way from Point Reyes on the south to the bluffs near Fort Ross on the north. Furlong Gulch lies immediately south, while the Russian River, Jenner, and Penny Island are visible in the middle distance to the north.

Returning the way you came, you rejoin the main loop trail at 2.8 miles. Although you could turn left and return the way you came, the described hike turns right and descends northeast through open grasslands towards Pomo Canyon Trail. (Both choices are nearly identical distances back to Shell Beach.) Cross a wooden footbridge at 2.9 miles and another hiker's gate through a wooden fence line at 3.0 miles. The descent steepens as you traverse a dense forest of chest-high coyote brush. Your next objective, Pomo Canyon Trail, is visible below to the left. Just as you enter a pine forest you reach the trail junction at 3.2 miles.

The trail to the right leads to Pomo Canyon Campground in 0.5 mile. If you choose this route, you will traverse a second-growth redwood forest with many excellent examples of fairy rings—mature trees that have sprouted around the base of a previously logged stump.

The described trail turns left and follows Pomo Canyon Trail west toward Shell Beach. At 3.4 miles you cross a plank bridge and begin climbing. Almost immediately a rough volunteer trail branches to the top of a small hill on your right. Other volunteer trails enter and leave as you continue on.

You exit the forest at 3.5 miles and start a descent. Thick stands of coastal hedge nettle grow alongside the trail here, with masses of purple flowers in the summertime. At 3.6 miles you climb through a mixed forest of redwood, bay, and big-leaf maple. Sword ferns and leather ferns line the slopes of a seasonal stream. The trail levels, then descends, at 3.7 miles, where a large redwood lies fallen across the path. Trail crews have cut an opening through the log.

At 3.9 miles you pass an ancient telephone pole and walk beside a forest of poison oak along an old fence line to the left. Keep children close at hand through this section. The trail alternately climbs and descends for the next mile. At 4.6 miles a side trail to your right leads to a picnic table at the top of a knoll. You again reach the junction with Red Hill trail at 4.9 miles. Keep right, following your original path in reverse, as you make the long final descent back to the trailhead at 5.4 miles and the Shell Beach parking lot at 5.5 miles.

Trail 10: Islands in the Sky Vista Loop Trail

Length: 4.1 miles round trip including side trip to Fern Tree Viewpoint, 2.5 hours

Difficulty: Strenuous

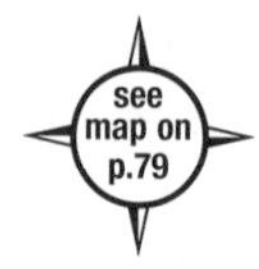

Overview: This trail is part of the upper Willow Creek acquisition that became part of Sonoma Coast State Park in 2005. The State currently lacks the funding to open it to the general public, so it is only accessible to holders of permits issued by LandPaths. Please note that unless you have a permit or are accompanied by a permit holder, you cannot take this trip. For more information, refer to their website at www.LandPaths.org.

This strenuous trail climbs 900 feet from the parking area through mixed redwood and Douglas-fir forest to a ridgeline with outstanding views of the coast. At the top, a short side trail leads to a unique "fern tree," a Douglas-fir with a large fern growing along one of its branches. In addition to the described hike, you can explore numerous other side trails. Some of these lead to private property, so study the map ahead of time to become familiar with the park boundaries. When on the trail, pay attention to posted signs.

Directions to Trailhead: Take Highway 116 to the town of Duncans Mills. Turn south on Moscow Road, cross the highway bridge, and immediately turn right onto Freezeout Road. Drive 0.3 mile to the second gate on the left. Permit holders are able to unlock the gate and drive 0.4 mile to the grass parking area. Automobiles should park on the left, diagonally to the entrance road. Horse trailers should park in the large open area to the right. Private vehicles are not permitted beyond the trailhead.

Trail Description: The trail is a broad, former logging road that starts at the south end of the parking area. You begin a steady climb through a forest of redwoods, Douglas-firs, and bay trees. The understory includes sword ferns, tanoaks, miner's lettuce, and redwood sorrel. Be alert for poison oak beside the trail.

You quickly reach a locked gate on your left leading to private property. Keep right, continuing the steady climb up the west side of Freezeout Creek. For much of the year you can hear the sound of running water far below. You can also look down to a clearing on private property and see the remains of an old picnic ground.

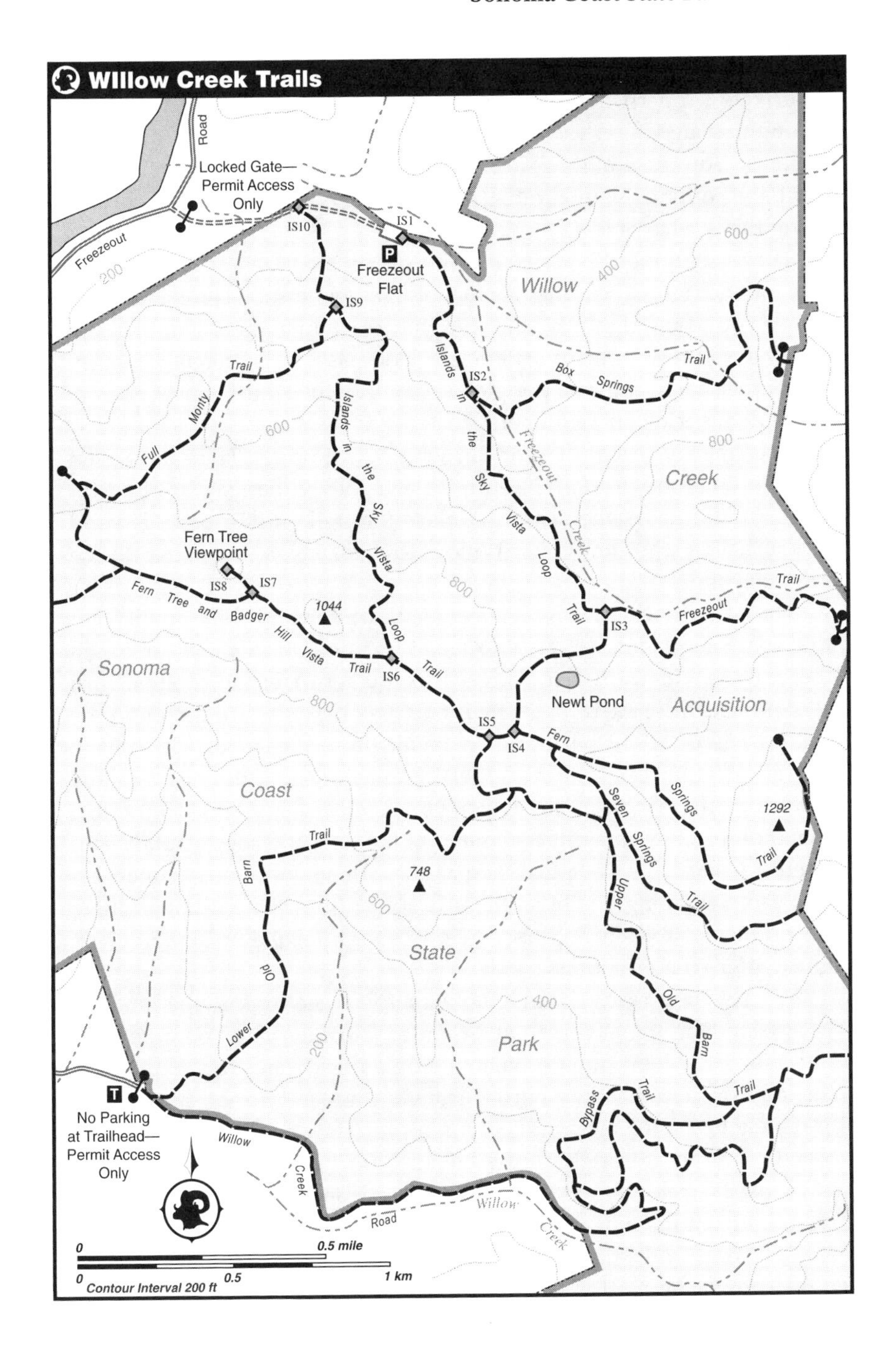
Willow Creek Trails
Road
Locked Gate—
Permit Access
Only
Freezeout
200
IS10
IS1
Freezeout
Flat
Willow
400
600
IS9
Trail
Full
Monty
Islands
in
the
Sky
Vista
Loop
Trail
IS2
Box
Springs
Trail
Freezeout
Creek
800
Creek
Fern Tree
Viewpoint
IS8
IS7
Fern
Tree
and
Badger
Hill
Vista
Trail
1044
IS6
IS3
Freezeout
Trail
Newt Pond
Sonoma
Acquisition
IS5
IS4
Fern
Springs
Trail
Seven
Springs
Trail
1292
Coast
Trail
Barn
748
Upper
State
Old
Barn
Old
Lower
Park
Bypass
Trail
Trail
No Parking
at Trailhead—
Permit Access
Only
Willow
Creek
Road
Willow
Creek
0
0.5 mile
0
0.5
1 km
Contour Interval 200 ft

At 0.5 mile you reach a second junction with another road leading to private property on your left. Keep right and continue the climb through shaded forest. The ascent briefly levels at 0.9 mile but soon resumes. You reach a third side road on your left at 1.0 mile. Stay to the right and continue your climb, still in forest. Look for flowering currant along this stretch of trail.

The forest thins at 1.2 miles as you pass an old road and a large dead snag on the right. The remains of an old gravel pit soon come into view below you to the right. By 1.4 miles you reach open grassland, having climbed 900 feet from the trailhead. Douglas iris, buttercups, scarlet pimpernel, and California poppies are some of the wildflowers you may see here in spring and summer.

You quickly reach the junction with Fern Springs Trail and Seven Springs Trail on your left. Keep right and follow the main trail northwest. An old fence line nearly parallels the trail on the south. Beyond it, you have great views over Willow Creek Canyon and across to the ridge beyond.

The junction with Old Barn Loop Trail, an interesting hike you'll want to save for another day, is on your left at 1.5 miles. At 1.7 miles you reach the junction with the trail to Badger Hill and Fern Tree viewpoints. Turn left and take this side trail northwest across open grassland, around the south flank of a first peak and on toward a second peak. The trail to Badger Hill viewpoint heads left at 2.0 miles. Keep right and continue toward Fern Tree viewpoint, which you reach at 2.1 miles. At 1,000 feet elevation you have magnificent views to the west and south, but the real interest is Fern Tree, a large Douglas-fir with an enormous leather-leaf fern growing along one of its massive lower branches. Although there are no picnic tables here, this is a good spot to take a break and enjoy lunch after your strenuous climb.

When you're ready, return the way you came back to the junction with Islands in the Sky Trail at 2.6 miles. Turn left and continue your trek along the loop, now a narrow single-track trail. You soon begin the long descent, heading north through grassland. In the spring, you are likely to see the rare sand crocus, a pink flower with six petals and a yellow center, throughout the hillside. To the north, Duncans Mills is visible far below. Just after you cross a seasonal creek at 2.8 miles, the road from the gravel pit joins on your right. You reenter the mixed forest of redwoods, firs, wild rose, and poison oak at 2.9 miles. As you travel down the west side of an unnamed gulley, the forest thickens and the understory teems with sword ferns, wood ferns, Douglas iris, milkmaids, and wild rose.

At 3.1 miles you pass a car-size boulder that recently tumbled from the side of the hill onto the trail. Continuing your descent, the trail skirts the transition between grassland and forest before reentering the forest of firs, tanoaks, and an occasional bay tree at 3.3 miles. You reach the junction with Full Monty Trail at 3.6 miles, where in the spring, you may see a miniature forest of distinctive powder-blue flowers with white centers known as Pacific hound's tongue. Keep right and continue descending. Use caution, as several springs along here keep the adobe trail wet and slippery throughout the rainy season.

The descent ends at 3.8 miles as you reach the road you drove in on. Turn right and follow this road back to the trailhead at 4.1 miles. When you drive out, be sure to close and lock the gate behind you at Freezeout Road.

Trail 10: Islands in the Sky Vista Loop Waypoints (WGS84 Datum)

Name	Latitude	Longitude	Feature
IS1	N38° 26.885′	W123° 02.507′	Trailhead at parking lot
IS2	N38° 26.612′	W123° 02.341′	Junction with 1st road to private property on left
IS3	N38° 26.245′	W123° 02.054′	Junction with 2nd road to private property on left
IS4	N38° 26.032′	W123° 02.262′	Junction with Fern Springs and Seven Springs Trails
IS5	N38° 26.033′	W123° 02.311′	Junction with Old Barn Trail
IS6	N38° 26.167′	W123° 02.517′	Junction with Badger Hill and Fern Tree Viewpoint Trails
IS7	N38° 26.280′	W123° 02.833′	Badger Hill Trail/Fern Tree Trail divergence point
IS8	N38° 26.329′	W123° 02.896′	Fern Tree Viewpoint
IS9	N38° 26.770′	W123° 02.658′	Junction with Full Monty Trail
IS10	N38° 26.959′	W123° 02.739′	Junction with road. Turn right to return to trailhead.

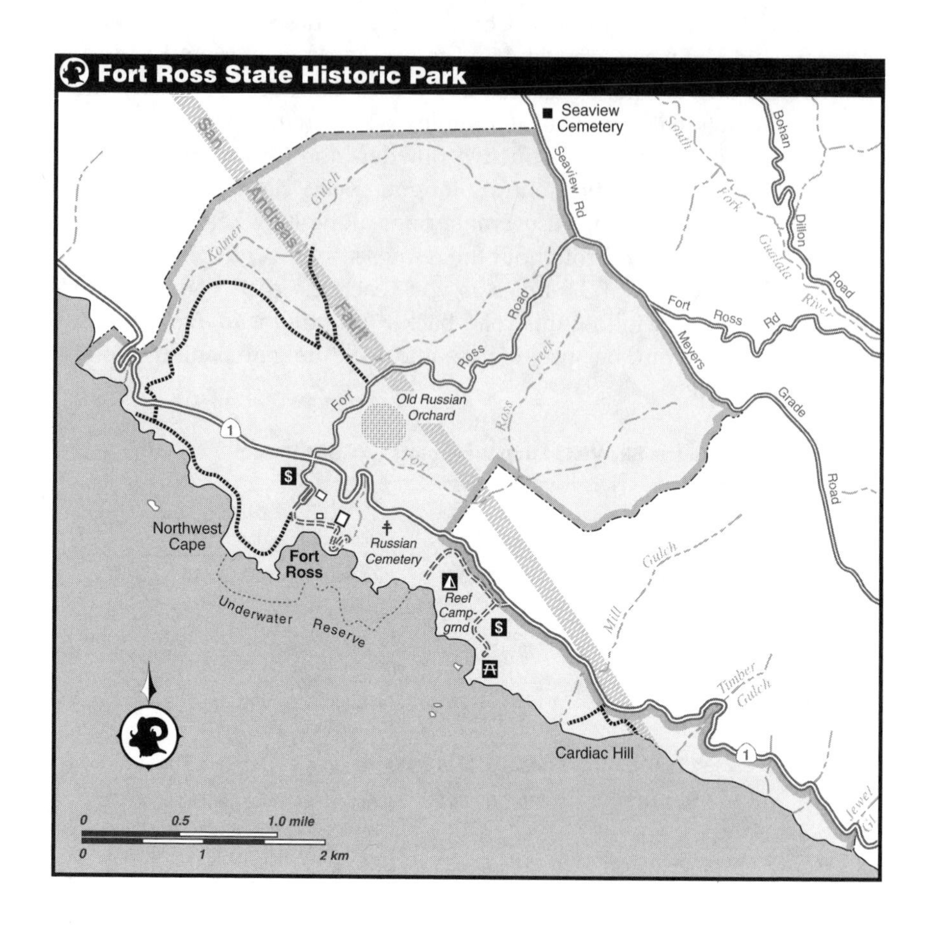

Fort Ross State Historic Park
Seaview Cemetery
Seaview Rd
South Fork Gualala River
Bohan Dillon Road
San Andreas Fault
Kolmer Gulch
Fort Ross Road
Fort Ross Rd
Meyers Grade Road
Ross Creek
Old Russian Orchard
Fort Ross Creek
1
Northwest Cape
Fort Ross
Russian Cemetery
Reef Camp-grnd
Underwater Reserve
Mill Gulch
Timber Gulch
Cardiac Hill
Jewel Gl
0
0.5
1.0 mile
0
1
2 km

Chapter 3

Fort Ross State Historic Park

The weathered remains of California's first permanent coastal settlement north of San Francisco stand on a grassy bluff overlooking the ocean at Fort Ross. It was here in 1812 that Russian colonists established the southernmost outpost of their Pacific empire and very nearly changed the course of history. If not for a few twists of fate, what we now call Sonoma County might today be part of a Russian colony stretching from Alaska to the Golden Gate. But such was not to be, and the reconstructed fort now stands as a silent reminder of the harshness of pioneer life in a strange and isolated land.

The historic stockade is the centerpiece of 3,303-acre Fort Ross State Historic Park. Here, you can explore the grounds and learn what life was like during the Russian era. Other points of interest include a visitor center, a 20-site campground, day-use areas, ocean access, an underwater park, an orchard and cemetery dating back to Russian times, and the Stanley S. Spyra Memorial Redwood Grove. The San Andreas Fault also passes through the park. Although there are no designated hiking trails, there are several informal paths and you are welcome to roam about the entire park. Remember to watch for poison oak when exploring the countryside!

The park sponsors a Cultural Heritage Day on the last Saturday of July each year. Over 100 volunteers dress in period costumes to depict a typical day in the life of the Ross Colony of the early 19th century. Visitors can watch a blacksmith at work, learn how to weave baskets, and listen to musicians playing traditional Russian music. Several times during the day, costumed participants recreate historic events such as visits from Spanish authorities or Yankee traders. A highlight of the day is the firing of the park's muzzle-loading cannons.

Archaeologists from the State and several universities still excavate within the park. One major objective is to understand more about how Russian colonialism impacted the native Pomo people. Recent explorations have not only included work inside the fort compound, but also in the cemetery, the surrounding neighborhoods, and in the cove below the fort, where timbers have been excavated from a shipway used to

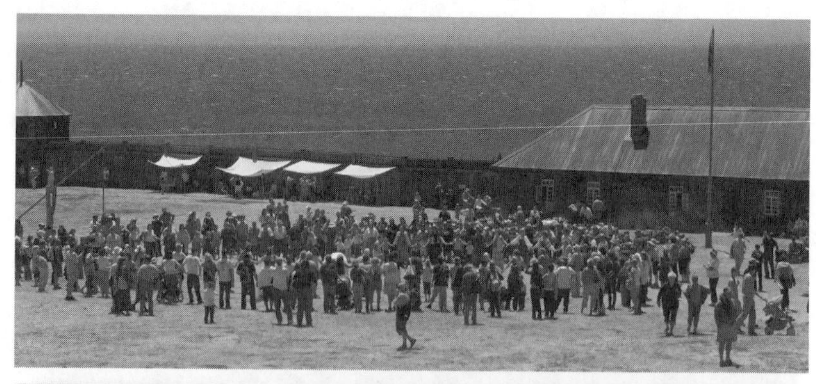

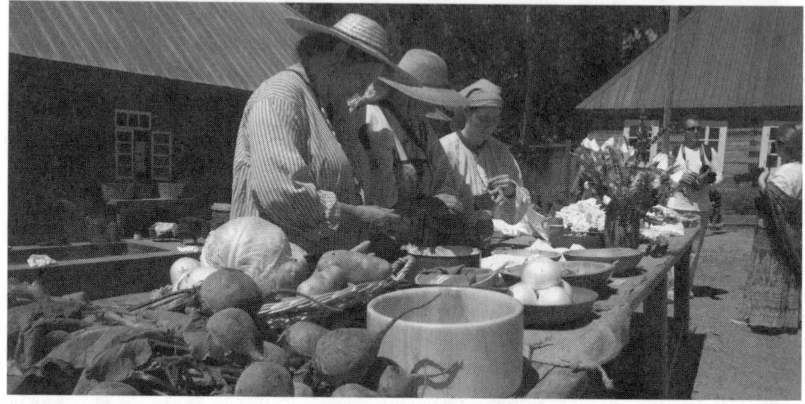

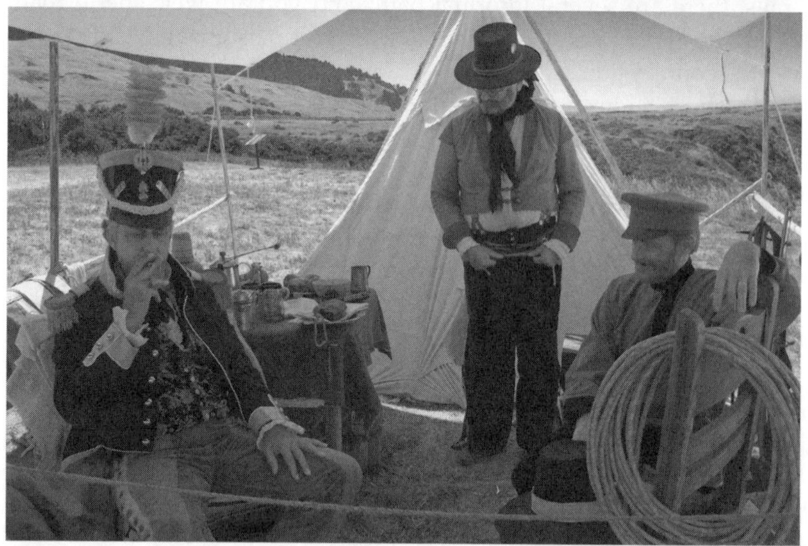

History comes alive at the Fort Ross Cultural Heritage Day, held on the last weekend of July each year.

launch vessels constructed at the site. Remember that all archaeological relics within the park are protected and must not be disturbed.

Getting There

The park lies 12 miles north of Jenner on State Highway 1. You come to the campground and day-use areas first, with the fort another 1.7 miles beyond.

The narrow, winding road out of Jenner quickly climbs as high as 600 feet above the sea, with sheer drops on your left. Passengers have excellent views of the rugged Sonoma Lost Coast along the way, but the driver will be too busy trying to stay on the road to appreciate them. Stop at any of the dirt pullouts alongside the road to enjoy the scenery. Also be sure to watch out for cattle that occasionally meander onto the highway.

Natural Environment

The fort stands on open grassland along a coastal shelf. To its east lies a range of hills that alternate between redwood-forested canyons and exposed ridges. The San Andreas Fault runs along the base of these hills less than a mile from the fort. If you explore within the rift zone you will see ample evidence of geologic activity. Fault trenches and sag ponds are especially evident in the area near Kolmer Gulch.

The park harbors a rich variety of wildlife. Common animals include the black-tailed deer, brush rabbit, ground squirrel, raccoon, pocket gopher, and broad-handed mole. You may also be lucky enough to spot the elusive bobcat or gray fox. Mountain lions have occasionally been

View of Fort Ross from the Russian orchard.

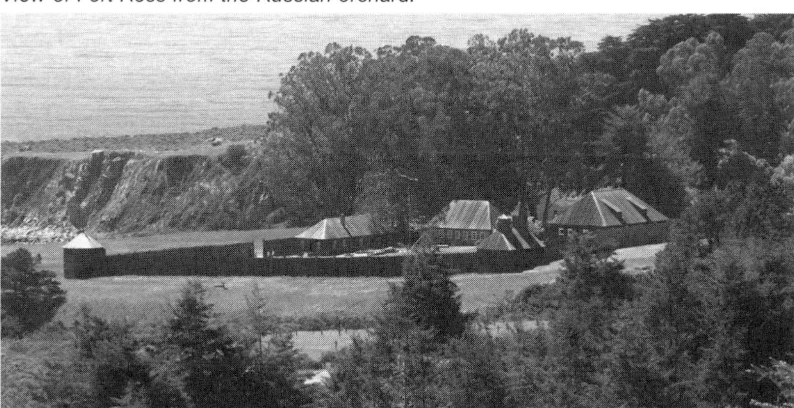

observed in the area, while black bear sightings are extremely rare. Numerous species of birds frequent the park, including hawks, ospreys, harriers, kestrels, and an assortment of sea birds.

The weather here is typical of the Sonoma Coast. Summer highs are commonly 60–80°F, cooling into the 50s at night. The habitual morning fogs and afternoon winds make it seem colder. Spring, with its beautiful wildflower displays and less frequent fog, is an especially good time to visit.

History

Humans have lived in the Fort Ross area for at least 7,000 years. At the time of European contact in the 1700s, the region around Fort Ross was the domain of the Pomo Indians. The Pomo were not a tribe in the classical sense, nor were they nomadic like the Indians of the Great Plains. Rather, they lived in localized bands, each consisting of no more than a few hundred people. Each band had its own territory that was fiercely protected. Dozens of bands lived in relative harmony throughout what is now Sonoma County. Those in the Fort Ross area were known as the Kashaya Pomo.

Amid such fertile surroundings, the Kashaya had little need for agriculture. From the shore, they harvested abalone, mussels, fish, crabs, and marine mammals. From the inland areas they hunted deer, elk, and numerous smaller animals. They also gathered a bountiful supply of nuts, berries, seeds, greens, and vegetables. During the summer months, they lived along the coast, while in the fall, they moved inland to warmer, more protected settlements. Although primarily hunter-gatherers, they did grow tobacco and farmed many native grasses for daily use.

The Russians were drawn to this region in search of sea otter pelts for their lucrative fur trade with the Orient. Their eastward expansion through Siberia and beyond paralleled America's push westward. As the English were settling New England, Russian fur hunters reached the Pacific Ocean. They began exploring the Aleutians in the middle of the 18th century and by 1784 had established outposts all the way to Kodiak Island.

In 1799, based on glowing reports from the east, Czar Paul granted the Russian-American Company exclusive rights to hunt furs from Siberia to the Alaskan mainland. Facing high expectations, Aleksandr Baranov, the governor of the Russian American Company colonies at the Alaskan outpost of Fort Alexander, struggled to make the venture as profitable as his superiors had led the Czar to believe. The Alaskan climate was harsh, and many of the settlers were unwilling serfs. Most did not take even the most elementary sanitary precautions, so sickness was a constant problem.

For years, Baranov had tried to improve conditions at the Alaskan colony. He instituted military discipline and improved relations with the local natives. In 1799 he led an expedition to establish a new outpost at Sitka. Morale gradually improved, but the colonists were poor farmers so the food shortages continued. To make matters worse, the Sitka outpost was nearly wiped out in an 1802 Tlingit Indian uprising.

In 1805, the head of the Russian-American Company, Nikolai Petrovich Rezanov, sailed into Sitka. Although the 42-year-old Russian nobleman had been a company official for 10 years, he had never before visited the Alaskan colonies. The dilapidated shacks and starving colonists he found were a stark contrast to the prosperous settlements described in dispatches. Baranov offered to resign on the spot, but Rezanov would have none of it. The two discussed the situation and soon agreed that the answer to their problems lay in southern expansion.

Rezanov led an expedition to San Francisco in the spring of 1806. His scurvy-ridden crew was in desperate straits as they sailed through

Wooden crosses mark the Russian cemetery on a hill overlooking the fort.

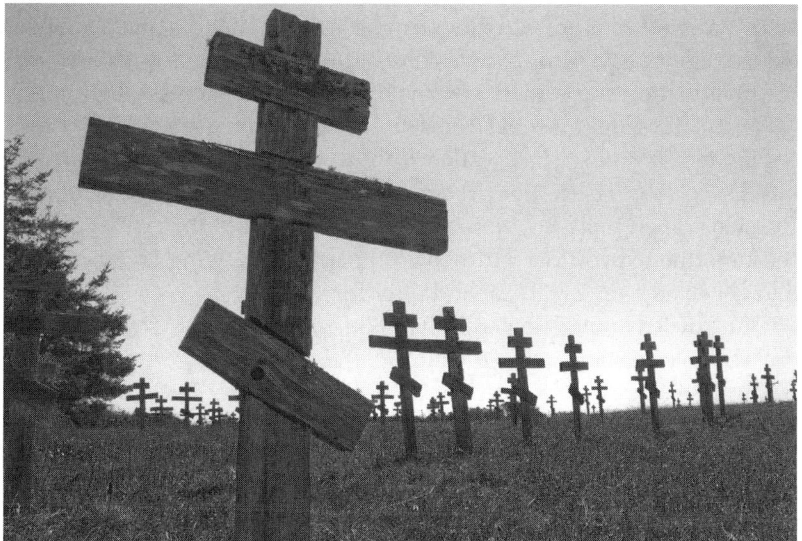

the Golden Gate on April 5. But the erudite Rezanov soon won over the suspicious Spaniards. He entered into a profitable trade arrangement in which the Russians received much-needed food in exchange for fine silks and other supplies.

Rezanov also courted María de la Conceptión Argüello y Moraga, the beautiful and charming 16-year-old daughter of the military commander. The two became engaged on condition that Rezanov, a Russian Orthodox, first return to St. Petersburg and receive papal dispensation to marry the Catholic María.

Rezanov left for Sitka on May 21, promising María he would return within two years. By February, 1807, he was in Siberia, ill with malaria but determined to reach St. Petersburg as quickly as possible. But while riding hard across the icy plains, he was killed when he fainted and fell from his horse. Years passed before María learned of Rezanov's death. Never marrying, she became a nun (the first in California) and lived in solitude until her death in 1857. Her plight was immortalized in a famous Bret Harte poem.

Had Rezanov returned to wed María, it could have altered the course of California history. United by marriage, Spain and Russia would have become formidable trading partners with an iron hold on the land. But with his death, so too died the dreams of a Russo-Spanish alliance, and the Spaniards returned to once again viewing the Russians as unwanted foreigners.

Rezanov, when he returned to Sitka in 1806, had urged Baranov to establish a hunting and farming colony north of San Francisco. So in 1808, Baranov sent an expedition under the command of Ivan Kuskov to search out a site. Kuskov[1] was one of the few men in the colony with the imagination and initiative to make the venture successful.

Forty Russians and 150 Native Alaskan Koniag and Aleut hunters landed in Bodega Bay (called Rumiantzev Bay by the Russians) in late December. The native Alaskan hunters, sailing small kayaks the Russians called *baidarkas*, were phenomenally successful in the hunt. By the time the expedition returned to Sitka the following October, they had collected over 2,000 seal and otter furs.

Kuskov led another expedition to Bodega Bay in 1811. They explored the countryside and traveled far up the Russian River, which they named the *Slavianka* (often translated as "Charming Little Slav Girl"). By now the Spanish were alerted to the Russian presence, but their

1 Popular historians frequently describe Kuskov as being peg-legged, although according to the Fort Ross Historical Society, there is no reliable evidence to support that theory.

small detachment was too weak to evict them. Once again, the Russians returned to Sitka with a bountiful harvest of furs.

These expeditions were so successful that Baranov sent Kuskov, along with 25 Russians and 80 Native Alaskans, back again to found a permanent colony in 1812. Kuskov decided that Bodega Bay was too close to San Francisco to be adequately defended, so he selected a spot about 18 miles farther north. The site had better soil, water, and pastureland, although its small cove was unable to accommodate large ships. Kuskov negotiated with the local Kashaya Pomo to purchase the land. According to accounts of the time, the purchase price was "three blankets, three pairs of breeches, two axes, three hoes, and some beads." Hardly a princely sum, but it was the only known instance during California's Spanish period in which land was actually purchased from the natives rather than simply taken from them.

Uncertain of Spanish intentions, the colonists immediately erected the 13-foot-high stockade walls. Around the fort and in the blockhouses at the north and south corners, as many as 40 cannons—some captured during Napoleon's retreat from Moscow—guarded the surroundings. Other buildings eventually erected within the fort included barracks, storehouses, a manager's house, and a chapel. Most of the Russian colonists lived in a settlement, or *sloboda,* outside the fort, near the native Alaskans and a village of Kashaya Pomo. Bodega Bay, with its better harbor, remained the colony's principal port.

The settlement, named Rossiya after the ancient name for the Russian homeland, was dedicated on August 13, 1812. To the Spanish, it became known as "Fuerto de los Rusos," while the Americans simply called it "Fort Ross."

Officially, both Spain and the United States viewed the Russian outpost with alarm. President James Monroe even issued his famous Monroe Doctrine in part to warn the Russians to depart. But the local Spaniards were generally willing to look the other way. San Francisco was a lonely and isolated outpost, so the prospect of meeting interesting foreigners was appealing. Clandestine trading was common, and in later years—after 1822—Mexican officials were sometimes invited to ceremonial events at the fort.

The abundance of nearby timber encouraged company officials to set up a shipyard in the cove below the fort, the first in California. Vasilli Grudiinin, a master shipbuilder sent from Sitka, struggled to build sturdy ships using unfamiliar local tanoak. Over a period of eight years three large brigs, a schooner, and several smaller ships were built and launched from the site. But the wood quickly rotted, making them

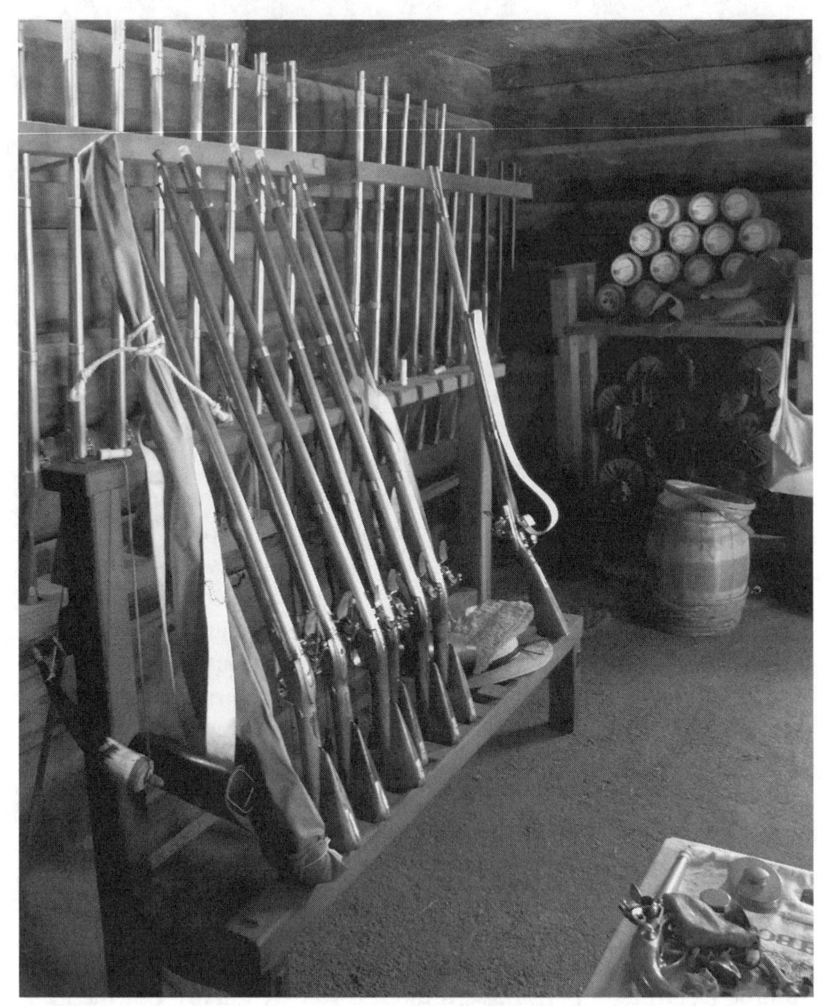

The armory at the Kuskov House is maintained much the way it may have looked in Russian times, including these replicas of period muskets.

suitable only for coastal trade. Many of the smaller ships found a ready market among the local Spanish settlers.

The fort also gave Russian scientists a base to study the flora and fauna of the north coast. On one visit, the Russian naturalist Adelbert von Chamisso collected samples of the California poppy. He gave it the scientific name *Eschscholtzia Californica* after his friend and fellow traveler, the entomologist Johan Eschscholtz. Later, the governor-general of Russian America, Baron Ferdinand von Wrangell, led a major anthropological study of Indian tribes in the Sonoma County area.

The fear and strife so common elsewhere between Indians and Europeans did not exist at Fort Ross because the Russians treated the Kashaya with relative fairness. Indians were paid in flour and meat for their work, as well as with lodging and clothing. They were not held against their will, and many Russian and Alaskan men married Kashaya women, creating a unique tri-cultural community.

In the early years, the fur harvest was profitable, but by the 1820s overharvesting had decimated the sea otter population. So the colony turned to agriculture and livestock-raising as the dominant occupations. The old Russian orchard on the east side of Highway 1 survives as a remnant of this effort. But the colony was never successful enough to significantly help the Alaskan outposts. The colonists considered themselves hunters rather than farmers, so they never spent the time necessary to learn the finer points of farming. That, coupled with problems of gophers, mice, and coastal fog, doomed their efforts. Debts mounted year by year, and eventually the Russians were forced to withdraw. They unsuccessfully tried to sell the fort in turn to the Hudson's Bay Company, France, Mariano Vallejo, and the Mexican government. Finally in 1841, they reached an agreement with Johann Sutter, of Sutter's Fort along the American River, for the sale of the buildings, livestock, and implements. (In a separate, secret deed that did not surface until 1857, they also sold him the land.) After the purchase, he dismantled many of the buildings and used them to help found the town of Sacramento.

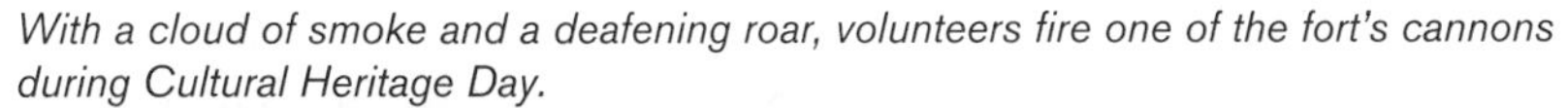

With a cloud of smoke and a deafening roar, volunteers fire one of the fort's cannons during Cultural Heritage Day.

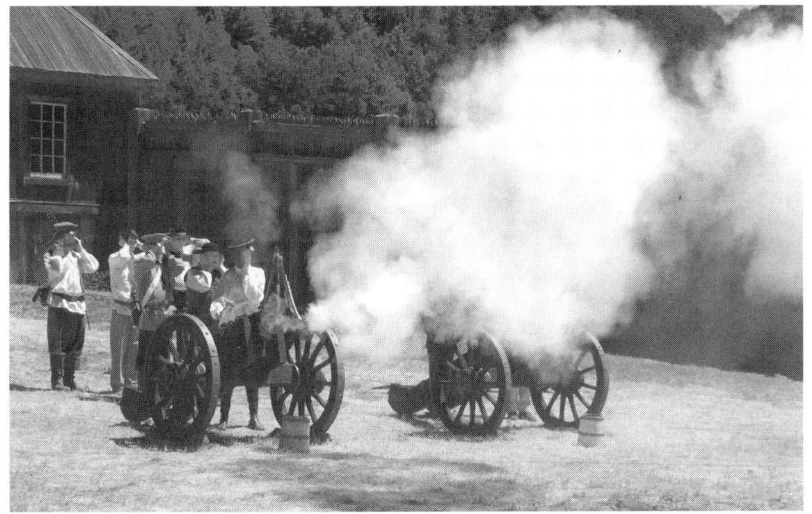

The Keys to the Fort

In July 2005, a long-forgotten relic of the Russian era returned to Fort Ross when John C. Benitz presented two massive iron keys to surprised rangers at the park. Housed in a small wooden box, one was labeled "main gate" and the other "Russian chapel." The keys had been in the Benitz family's possession since the time of William Otto Benitz, John Benitz's great-grandfather, who first came to manage the fort for Johann Sutter in 1843. William Benitz later leased and eventually purchased the fort and surrounding lands, living there until 1867, when he relocated with his family to Argentina.

The existence of the keys came as a surprise because there are no records that the fort ever had locks. Archaeologists have confirmed the keys to be of the Russian era, and given the Benitz family history, there is little doubt they are genuine. When presenting the keys to the State, John Benitz explained how they had been handed down through the generations, residing for years in a small museum in his mother's house. They are now proudly displayed in the much larger museum at the Fort Ross Visitor Center.

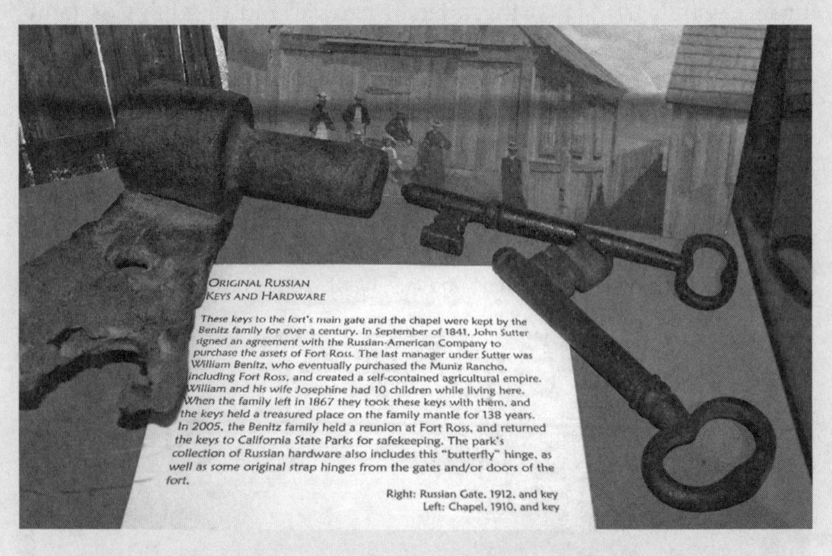

ORIGINAL RUSSIAN
KEYS AND HARDWARE
These keys to the fort's main gate and the chapel were kept by the Benitz family for over a century. In September of 1841, John Sutter signed an agreement with the Russian-American Company to purchase the assets of Fort Ross. The last manager under Sutter was William Benitz, who eventually purchased the Muniz Rancho, including Fort Ross, and created a self-contained agricultural empire. William and his wife Josephine had 10 children while living here. When the family left in 1867 they took these keys with them, and the keys held a treasured place on the family mantle for 138 years. In 2005, the Benitz family held a reunion at Fort Ross, and returned the keys to California State Parks for safekeeping. The park's collection of Russian hardware also includes this "butterfly" hinge, as well as some original strap hinges from the gates and/or doors of the fort.
Right: Russian Gate, 1912, and key
Left: Chapel, 1910, and key

After the Russians departed, Mexico rejected any claim Sutter had to the land and instead granted title to Manuel Torres. The fort changed hands several times in subsequent years until 1873, when it was purchased by George W. Call. Besides raising cattle, he also grew fruits and vegetables and conducted a profitable lumber-harvesting operation at the site. The Call family owned the fort as part of a 15,000-acre ranch until 1903, when they sold the fort and 3 acres of land to the California

Historical Landmarks Committee. By the time it was turned over to the State of California in March 1906, much of the original construction had deteriorated or had been removed. Less than a month later, the great San Francisco earthquake ravaged the fort. Over the years, the State has carried out extensive restoration work and has continued to add acreage, so that today the fort is similar to its appearance in the Russian period.

Stockade and Surroundings

Driving north on Highway 1, you'll catch your first glimpse of the fort walls while still 2 miles away. Unlike many historic sites now enveloped by commercial development, Fort Ross sits in an environment largely unchanged from Ivan Kuskov's day. In fact, thanks in part to careful preservation efforts by a number of people and organizations, the region is less developed now than it was during the Russian period.

As you drive past the fort, look for a driveway on your left leading to the stockade. This was the original route of Highway 1, which went right through the center of the compound until 1972, when it was relocated to its present route. You'll find the park's main entrance a short distance north, opposite the junction with Fort Ross Road. Stop at the kiosk to pay your entrance fee, then continue to the large parking lot at the visitor center. Here, you'll find an easy path to the fort. Along the trail, you'll pass numerous garden plots planted by elementary school children as part of an overnight outdoor education experience.

During the school year, Fort Ross serves as an overnight outdoor education site for elementary school children. These garden plots were planted by children serving in the role of agronomists.

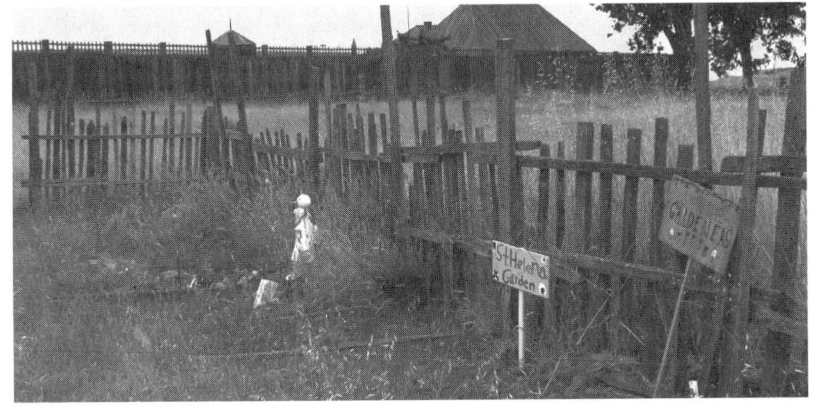

Many visitors seem to think they are done once they've toured the stockade. Don't fall into this trap; there is much to see beyond the fort walls. Several points of interest are easily accessible from the main parking lot.

Stockade

Few people realize that most of what you now see of the stockade is a reconstruction of the original. One exception is the Rotchev House, built in 1836 and now a registered National Historic Landmark. Only a few of the other structures that once stood here have been restored. The following structures now stand within the stockade walls.

Kuskov House. This two-story building was the original commandant's house. The upper story contained the living quarters while the lower story contained the armory and storerooms. After Alexander Rotchev moved the commandant's residence to new quarters, the Kuskov House may have provided lodging for scientists and other distinguished visitors who stayed for long periods.

Chapel. Nothing symbolizes the resilience of Fort Ross more that its simple wooden chapel. Built around 1824, it was the first Russian Orthodox Church in North America outside of Alaska. The hardy structure survived the ravages of time until 1906, when it collapsed during the great San Francisco earthquake. It could easily have been written off as irretrievably lost, but citizens' groups from around the State persevered. Finally in 1916 they convinced the State legislature to appropriate $3,000 for reconstruction. George Call's son, Carlos, supervised the

Kuskov House.

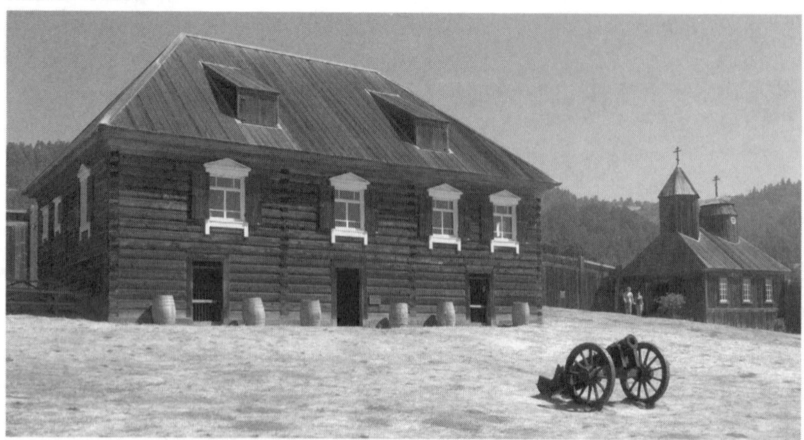

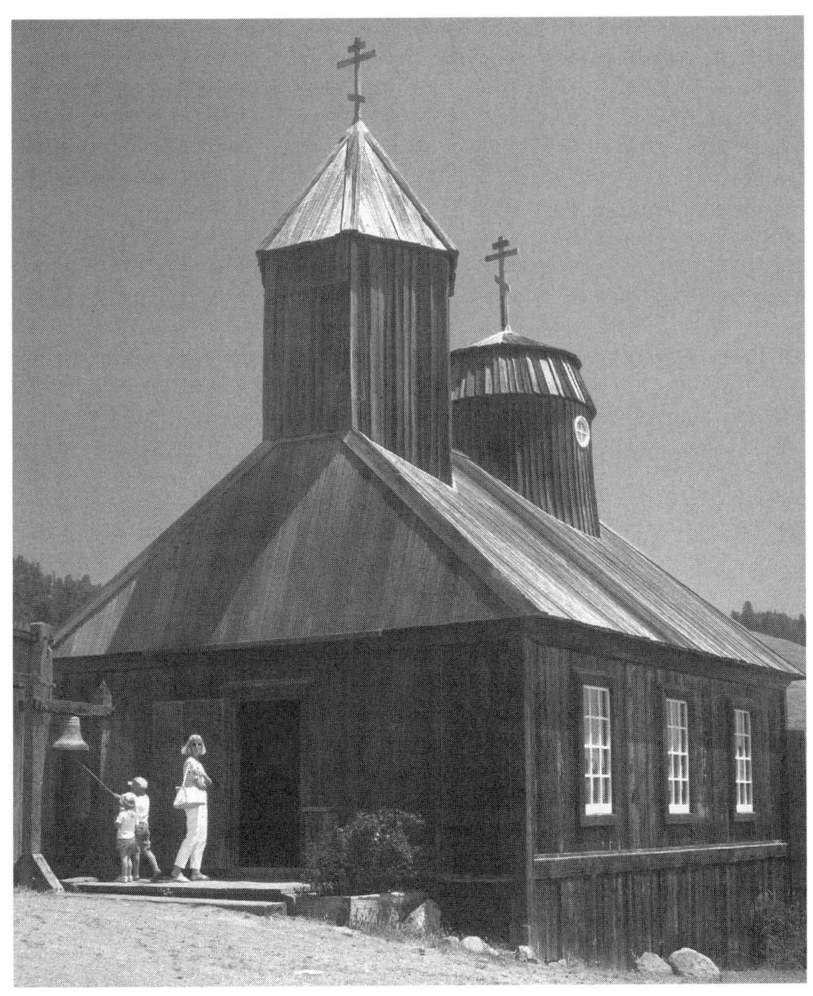

Chapel.

work. Fortunately, the roof, cupola, and bell tower were still intact, so most of the effort involved constructing new walls and foundations.

This reconstruction was not completely faithful to the original. To strengthen the walls, extra beams were added, so the number of side windows had to increase from three to four. There were also errors in the alignment with the stockade walls. Not until 1956 were most of these flaws corrected during a second restoration supervised by the park's historian, John C. McKenzie. His careful research and meticulous attention to detail were essential in assuring historical accuracy.

Another potentially fatal disaster occurred on October 5, 1970, when a fire of unknown origin burned the little chapel to the ground. Once again, supporters rallied to raise the funds to rebuild it. This time the reconstruction accurately duplicated the Russian original, including faithful reproductions of materials and construction techniques.

South Blockhouse. Part of the original stockade, the south blockhouse has eight sides. It guards the southeast and southwest walls, and its cannon could fire on ships at sea. It was partially rebuilt during the chapel's 1917 restoration and was completed by McKenzie in 1956–57.

Officials' Barracks. This structure, complete with kitchen and office, provided living accommodations for Russian officials and routine visitors. It also included storerooms, a jail, and workshops. During the late 1800s, its south end served as a saloon. The original timbers from the barracks were removed in 1917 and used to help reconstruct the chapel.

Rotchev House. Until Alexander Rotchev took over as the fort's final commander in 1836, no Russian women had lived in the commandant's house since Ivan Kuskov's departure 15 years earlier. When Rotchev

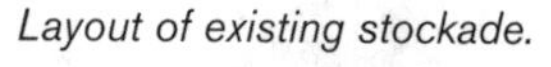
Layout of existing stockade.

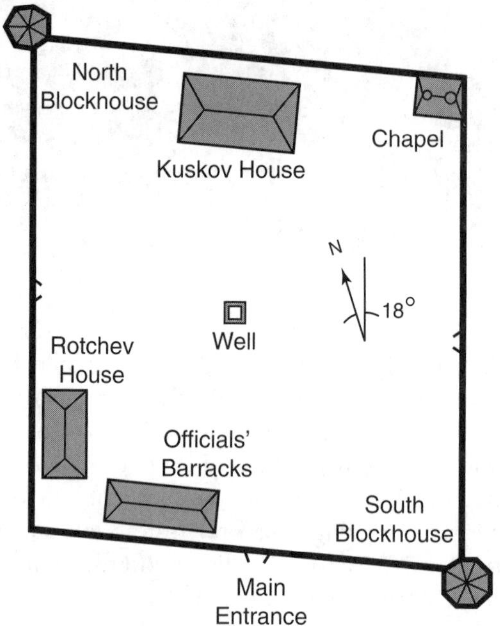

and his wife, the former Princess Helena Gagarina, arrived they immediately brought a new level of sophistication to the colony. But Helena was aghast at the idea of living in the Kuskov House above an arsenal full of explosive gunpowder. She immediately demanded new living quarters. The new residence, known as the Rotchev House, was located as far from the arsenal as possible.

After the Russians left, various owners made modifications to the house. William Benitz enlarged it for his family in 1847. He extended the building on the north and added a partial second story on the south. The Call family used it as a residence until completing their ranch house in 1878. It subsequently became a hotel before falling into disrepair. Restoration work began in 1925 and continued off and on for another half-century. The non-Russian additions were removed and various other repairs were carried out to restore its original appearance. Damaged by a fire in 1971, it was refurbished and opened to the public in 1974. The Rotchev House is the only surviving original structure from the Russian era and is one of the oldest wooden buildings west of the Mississippi. Its interior was recently refurbished with help from the Fort Ross Interpretive Association to portray living conditions typical of the early 19th century.

North Blockhouse. Unlike the south blockhouse, the north tower has only seven sides. It commands an unobstructed view over the northeast and northwest walls. After lying in disrepair for a number of years, it was ultimately rebuilt in 1948.

Well. At the center of the stockade lies a well capable of providing water even during siege. Opinions differ as to whether it or Fort Ross Creek was the colony's primary water source in routine times. The well has been shown to be one of the few reliable year-round water sources in the vicinity.

Additional Buildings. During the Russian period several additional buildings existed within the compound. These included a two-story warehouse north of the Rotchev House, a barracks for unmarried employees south of the chapel, and a warehouse/kitchen near the south blockhouse. There was also a large windmill, the first in California, northwest of the stockade. These structures have all long since disappeared, though park officials hope to eventually reconstruct some of them. The warehouse is currently in the planning stage, and students at St. Mary's College in Moraga are have done field research to identify the location of the windmill.

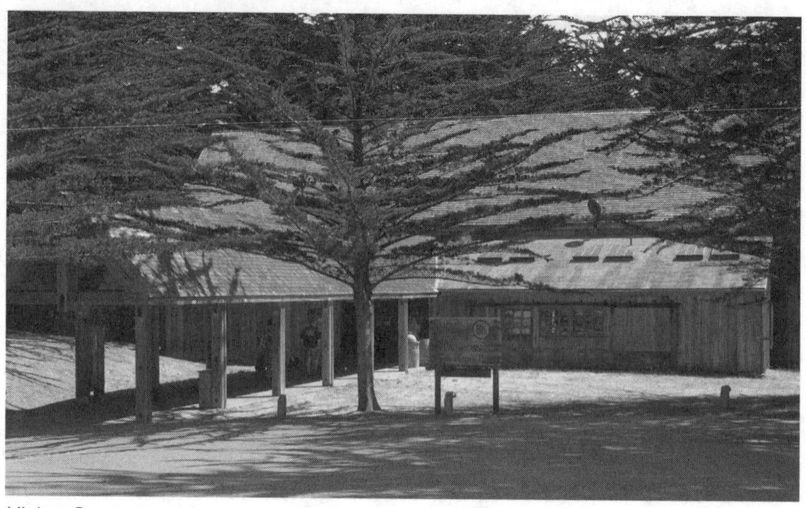

Visitor Center.

Visitor Center

Be sure to stop in at the visitor center before continuing on to the stockade. You'll find interpretive displays of the fort's history, a theater showing slide and video presentations related to the park, and a wide range of books and postcards for sale. Volunteers from the Fort Ross Interpretive Association staff the bookstore, whose proceeds are used to help fund research grants, maintain the old Russian orchard, restore buildings, and conduct the Environmental Living Program for elementary school children.

Call Ranch House and Picnic Area

After touring the stockade, exit through the southwest gate, opposite the Kuskov House. Follow the paved road as it bears right. For many years, this was the route of Highway 1. The wooden two-story ranch house stands on your right a few hundred feet from the fort. This was the house George W. Call built for his family in 1878. He also started a weather station here that is still in use today, making it the oldest weather station on the west coast. The ranch house is open for public tours 1–4 P.M. on the first weekend of each month.

Behind the house you can see a wooden barn, another relic from the Call period. Just past the ranch house is a picnic area with tables. From here, you can either turn right and follow a footpath through a picturesque grove of eucalyptus and Monterey cypress back to the visitor center or continue along the road back to the west end of the parking lot.

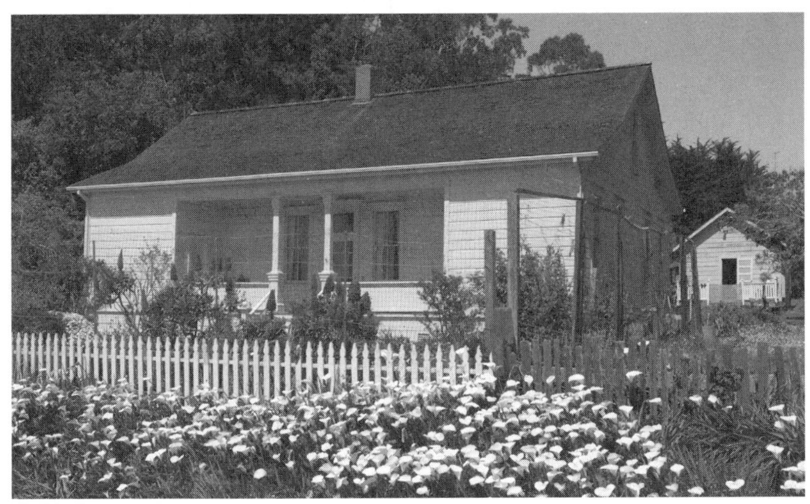

Call Ranch House.

Fort Ross Cove–Sandy Cove

From the stockade's main gate, take the access road south toward the sea. Follow it down the side of the cove to an excellent sandy beach with picnic tables. This is Sandy Cove, which was the industrial center of the Russian colony. It was here that the Russians set up California's first shipyard, as well as a tannery and blacksmith's shop. The remains of a wooden shipway and shipbuilding materials were excavated here in 1996–97 after being exposed by a winter storm.

To the north is Fort Ross Cove, a rocky cove that is good for tidepooling.

Underwater Park

The waters from Northwest Cape to Fort Ross Reef have been designated as an underwater park. Unlike the marine reserve at Salt Point State Park, you may still fish and dive for abalone here. However, as a park, it is afforded somewhat more protection than the surrounding waters.

Russian Cemetery

The old Russian cemetery stands on a grassy knoll across Fort Ross Creek from the stockade. The easiest access is from Highway 1 southeast of the fort. Park at a small gravel pullout near milepost 32.18, directly across from a gated dirt access road. Walk through an opening in the fence to the cemetery. You can also reach the cemetery by way of a quiet path east along a gully from Sandy Cove, as described on Page 105. The Russian Orthodox crosses marking the known burial sites are recent additions to replace the long-decayed original markers.

Along Fort Ross Road

Russian Orchard

You reach the orchard by driving along Fort Ross Road, which intersects Highway 1 directly across from the main park entrance. The orchard lies 0.5 mile up the road on the right. The trail through the orchard is described on Page 114.

The first trees planted by the Russians were peaches brought from San Francisco in 1814. Eventually, plantings were expanded to include hundreds of apple, cherry, and pear trees. Later, after the Russians' departure, William Benitz added another orchard across Fort Ross Road, although it is no longer extant. George W. Call used both orchards and planted many additional fruit trees.

The orchard continues in service today, with several of the original trees remaining. The Russians also planted grapes here, thereby earning the distinction of being Sonoma County's first vintners. Their lack

Several trees in the old orchard survive from Russian times.

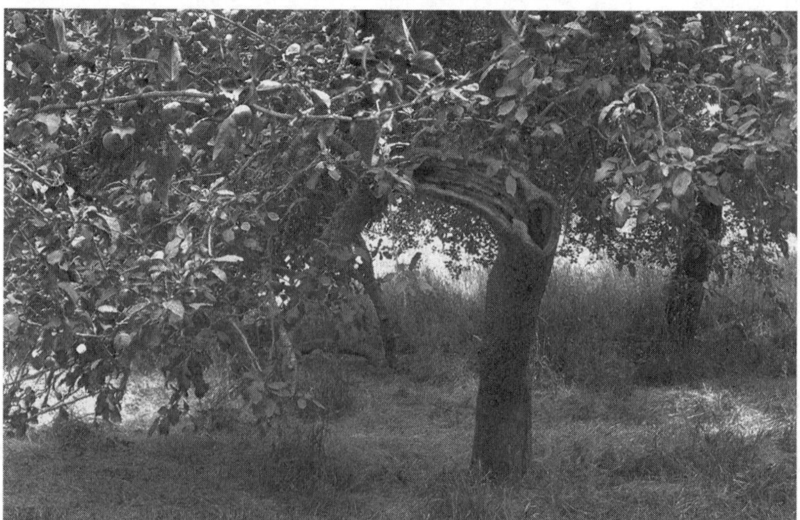

of success would hardly have foretold the region's future prospects as a center for fine wine.

Stanley S. Spyra Memorial Grove

This stately redwood grove lies nearly opposite the old orchard. The area was heavily logged beginning with the Russians and continuing with subsequent owners, so the trees here are now the world's oldest second-growth coast redwoods. A number of their trunks were broken during the 1906 earthquake when the ground moved more than 7 feet in less than a minute.

San Andreas Fault

The San Andreas rift zone passes just east of the stockade, running through the orchard and redwood grove. Ground movement over many centuries has caused portions of both Fort Ross Creek and Kolmer Gulch to turn parallel to the fault. You can see visible evidence of the fault by hiking the Kolmer Gulch Trail described on Page 108.

North Headlands

If your tastes run to hiking, wildlife observation, and coastal exploration, this is the area for you. You can start either at the fort's main

Fog and wind don't deter these picnickers from enjoying the headlands.

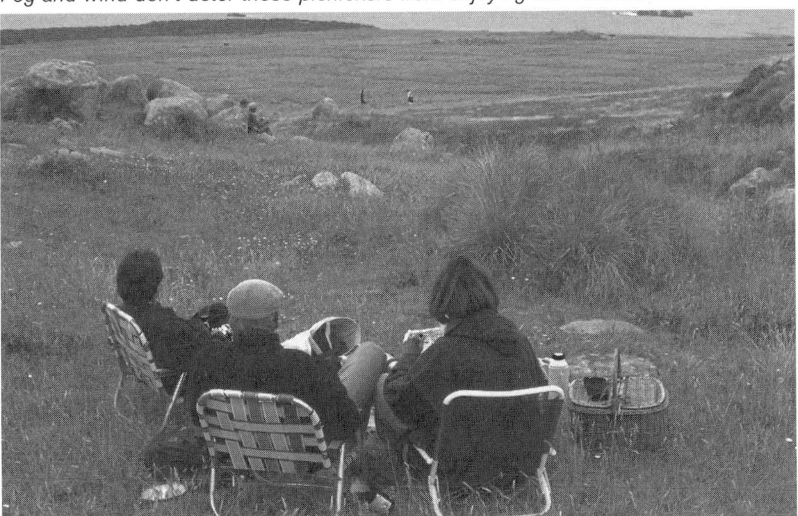

parking lot or at Windermere Point to explore the various trails that stretch out over the headlands. The North Headlands Trail is described in detail on Page 111.

Windermere Point

This jutting point at the north end of the park is named after a ship (spelled *Windemere* in some accounts) that wrecked here in 1883. Today, it provides ocean access to divers and fishermen. A rough dirt loop road departs west from the highway at the north side of the hairpin curve through Kolmer Gulch.

Reef Campground and Day-Use Areas

The only camping allowed in the park is at Fort Ross Reef Campground, set in a protected canyon southeast of the stockade. There are also two day-use areas here. Fees are charged both for camping and for day use.

Campground

The campground entrance is located along Highway 1 near milepost 31.37. Register at the kiosk and continue along the road to the campsites.

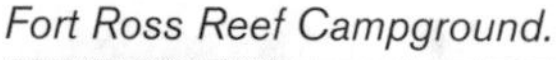

Fort Ross Reef Campground.

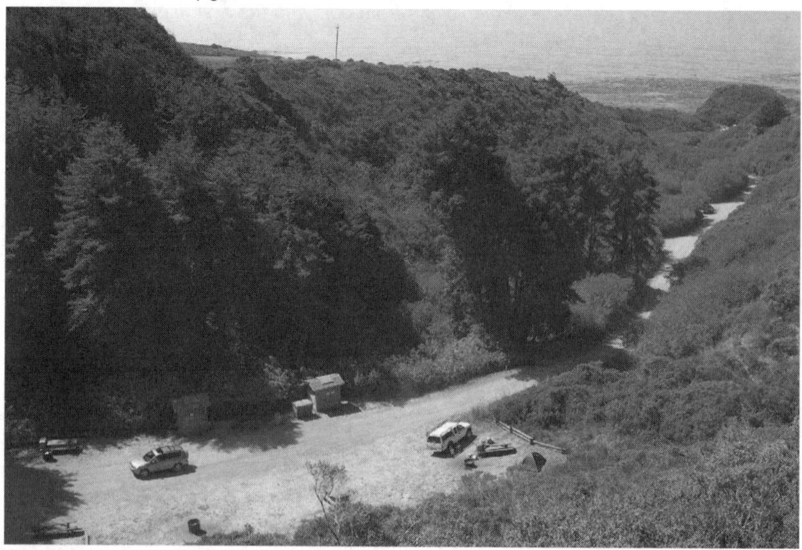

Open from April 1 to November 30, the campground contains 20 sites available on a first-come-first-served basis. Because of very limited turning space, the campground cannot accommodate large recreational vehicles. Each campsite includes a picnic table and fire ring. What look like primitive outhouses are actually comfortable restrooms with flush toilets, sinks, and water faucets. There are no showers. During periods of high fire danger, campfires are not allowed, so be sure to check posted signs.

Day-Use Areas

The northern day-use area lies at the end of the road past the campground. A relatively easy path at the south end of the parking lot leads to a coarse gravel beach. Another, longer path on the north end leads to a rocky shoreline. The northern trail is more difficult; the last 20 feet involve scrambling over boulders down a rocky gully to the sea.

The road to the southern day-use area lies immediately left of the entrance kiosk. After paying your fee, take the narrow dirt road 0.25 mile to the grassy parking area. A poor dirt trail leads 120 feet down to a coarse gravel beach whose upper reaches are covered in driftwood. The trail is steep and narrow over loose dirt, so use extreme caution during the descent.

The day-use areas are popular spots for abalone diving and tidepooling. A valid California fishing license is required for any person 16 years of age and older. The reef is also a favorite spot for surfers willing to brave the cold Pacific waters and rocky shoreline.

Fort Ross State Historic Park Hiking Trails

Although there are no official hiking trails at Fort Ross, several logging roads from the Call Ranch era serve as informal trails and you are welcome to roam throughout most of the park. The only restriction is the fire road across the highway from the cemetery. Since it is the access to the park's water supply and to cabins used by visiting archaeologists, it is off limits to the public.

Several relatively easy trails depart from the area around the fort. A paved, disabled-access path from the visitor center leads to the stockade. From here, you can go down to the cove at Sandy Beach and continue on to the Russian Cemetery. Nearby, the North Headlands Trail and Reef Campground Trail both traverse windswept bluffs along the ocean.

Kolmer Gulch Trail and Orchard Trail start from Fort Ross Road about a half mile east of the fort. Kolmer Gulch Trail is a pleasant hike through quiet forest along the San Andreas Fault, while Orchard Trail allows you to explore remnants of the old Russian orchard. Cardiac Hill, a short but steep descent to the sea about 2 miles south of the fort, is a popular ocean access for abalone divers.

As you explore the park, remember that all archaeological relics are protected by law. Also be sure to watch for poison oak when hiking the countryside!

Trail 11: Visitor Center to Stockade, Sandy Cove, and Cemetery

Length: 0.2 mile to stockade, 0.9 mile to cemetery

Difficulty: Easy, disabled accessible to stockade, moderate to Sandy Cove and Cemetery

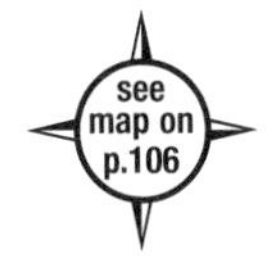

Overview: An easy, paved trail leads from the visitor center to the stockade. From there, you can take a gravel road down to the beach at Sandy Cove. Near the beach lies the junction with a quiet trail through mixed forest to the old Russian cemetery.

Directions to Trailhead: Take Highway 1 to the Fort Ross main entrance road. Turn west into the park, pay the entrance fee, and park at the east end of the lot near the visitor center.

Trail Description. Start by touring the visitor center, where you can learn the history of the fort, see relics of the past, watch video presentations, and purchase books and postcards related to the park. When finished, exit out the back door and down the steps. The trail to the fort, a paved path through a stand of cypress trees, is on your left. You cross a footbridge and emerge into open grassland at 0.1 mile. Several buildings from the Call Ranch era can be seen to your right, including a collapsed barn. The trail heads toward the northeast side of the stockade, directly toward the seven-sided North Blockhouse. The fenced-off garden plots on your right were planted by elementary school children as part of an overnight outdoor education experience.

When you reach the North Blockhouse the trail turns right and parallels the stockade's west wall, reaching the side entrance next to the Rotchev house at 0.2 mile. Enter here and tour the stockade and buildings within. Be sure to see the reconstructed armory inside the Kuskov House and additional exhibits inside the Rotchev House. You will also want to spend time inside the reconstructed chapel and the Officials' Barracks, and climb to look out the viewing ports of the blockhouses.

When finished touring the stockade, exit through the main entrance at the center of the south wall. Until 1972, this was the route of State Highway 1. As you exit the gate, look to your right to see the remains of the old highway heading north past the Call ranch house. Continue straight ahead. Your trail, now a wide gravel road, traverses the grassy bluffs toward the ocean. Be alert along here, as vehicles are allowed to

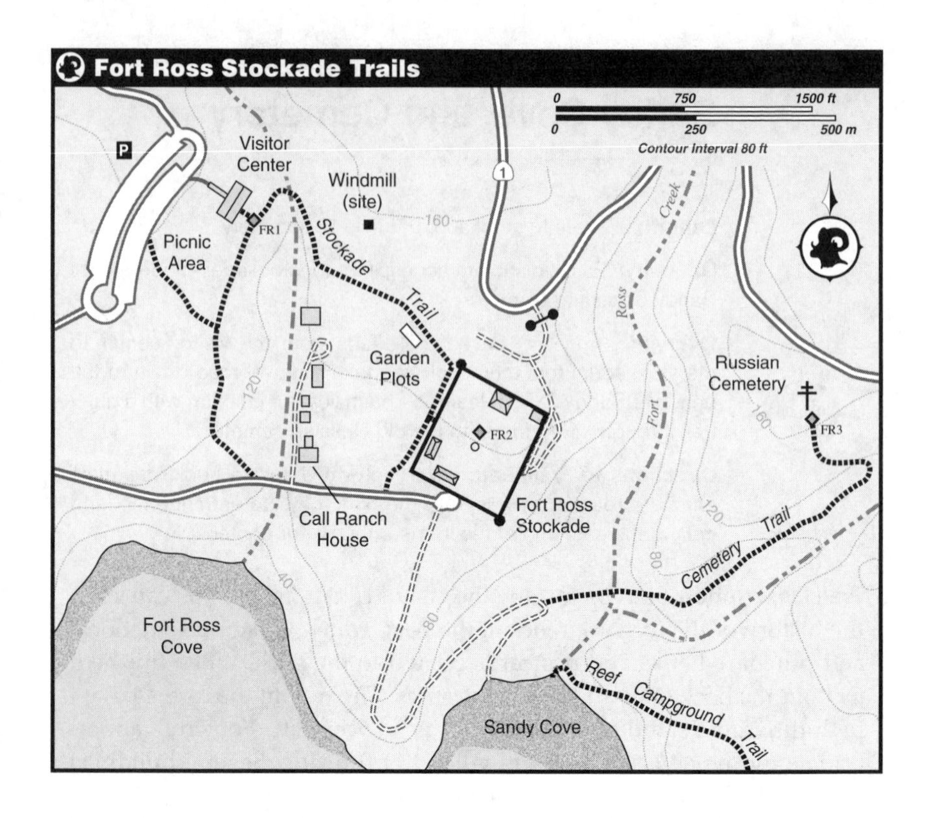

drive down to Sandy Cove long just long enough to drop off passengers and supplies before returning to the visitor center parking lot.

The trail curves sharply left 0.2 mile from the stockade and descends along the side of the bluff down to the beach. At 0.3 mile you reach Fort Ross Creek and on the left, the junction with the trail to the cemetery. It is just a short walk over to Sandy Cove, a nice beach that was a bustle of activity in the early 19th century. Spend some time there before returning to the cemetery trail junction.

At the junction, carefully cross Fort Ross Creek. The waters are usually shallow and you can rock-hop to stay dry. The narrow, overgrown trail climbs steadily up the left side of a tributary ravine of Fort Ross Creek, where you will see cow parsnip, yarrow, miners lettuce, giant vetch, wild blackberry, sword ferns, bracken ferns, and red elderberry. In the early spring, hounds tongue—a light blue flower with a white center—blooms profusely along the trail. Fir trees and oaks provide ample shade. Be sure to watch for poison oak along the trail.

At 0.5 mile you break out of the forest into open grassland to see Douglas iris, buttercups, and blue-eyed grass. An old fence line runs parallel to the trail on your right. A natural spring here keeps the trail wet and slippery through the rainy season. Near the top of the climb, you hike through a patch of chest-high coyote brush. The stockade is visible a few hundred yards to the west. The trail emerges onto the south side of the cemetery at 0.6 mile. An archaeological survey conducted here in the early 1990s identified over 150 burials at the site. The dozens of Russian orthodox markers you see today are modern crosses that have replaced the long-decayed original markers.

Highway 1 passes right beside the cemetery, and across the road is a gravel road leading into the hills. Until recently this path to Fort Ross Creek was open to hikers, but because it passes directly beside park maintenance facilities and a series of cottages reserved for visiting archaeologists, it is now closed to the general public.

When you are finished visiting the cemetery, return the way you came back to the stockade and visitor center, for a total round-trip distance of approximately 1.8 miles.

Trail 11 **Fort Ross Stockade Trails Waypoints (WGS84 Datum)**

Name	Latitude	Longitude	Feature
FR1	N38° 30.963′	W123° 14.774′	Fort Ross Visitor Center
FR2	N38° 30.851′	W123° 14.617′	Fort Ross Stockade
FR3	N38° 30.866′	W123° 14.411′	Russian Cemetery

Trail 12: Kolmer Gulch Trail

Length: 4.0 miles round trip to Lower Kolmer Gulch, 2.5 hours; 1.8 miles round trip to Kolmer Gulch Camp, 1 hour

Difficulty: Moderate

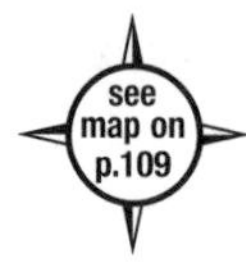

Overview: You can see evidence of the San Andreas fault by hiking an overgrown logging road from Fort Ross Road to Kolmer Gulch. Along the way, you pass through the Stanley S. Spyra Memorial Grove, the world's oldest second-growth redwood forest, then through open grasslands and mixed forest. Take the Upper Kolmer Gulch fork to reach Kolmer Gulch Camp, a secluded picnic area, or the Lower Kolmer Gulch fork to hike as far as Highway 1. Either direction offers plenty of solitude, and is a great hike for days when strong winds discourage you from hiking the exposed coastline.

Directions to Trailhead: Take Highway 1 to the Fort Ross main entrance road. Rather than turning west to the visitor center and stockade, turn east on Fort Ross Road. Drive 0.5 mile to a small turnout marking the grove entrance on your left, across the road from the Russian orchard. Park here, being careful not to block the fire access gate.

Trail Description: The trail begins just past the access gate into the redwood grove. As you walk the path, notice the fault trench to your left. The trail soon traverses the left edge of a large, reed-filled sag pond surrounded by horsetail ferns. Sag ponds occur when the ground sinks along the fault, forming an elongated depression that captures rainwater. Smaller ponds dry up by late summer, but this one is large enough to stay wet year round.

The trail forks at the far end of the sag pond. The right fork (impassible in the wet season) leads to Kolmer Gulch Camp, the left fork leads eventually to Highway 1. Take the left fork, marked LOWER KOLMER GULCH. You quickly emerge from the forest into open grassland. As you crest a slight rise, look down to your left to see another reed-filled sag pond. The road sweeps broadly left, then right, through rolling grasslands with views of the ocean. At 0.4 mile, you re-enter forest for most of the rest of your hike. The Call family logged the open forest here in the latter part of the 19th century. You can still see frequent stumps, now well over 100 years old. In the spring and early summer a profusion of wildflowers bloom along the trail. The foxglove, with its columns of pink bell-shaped flowers, is especially striking.

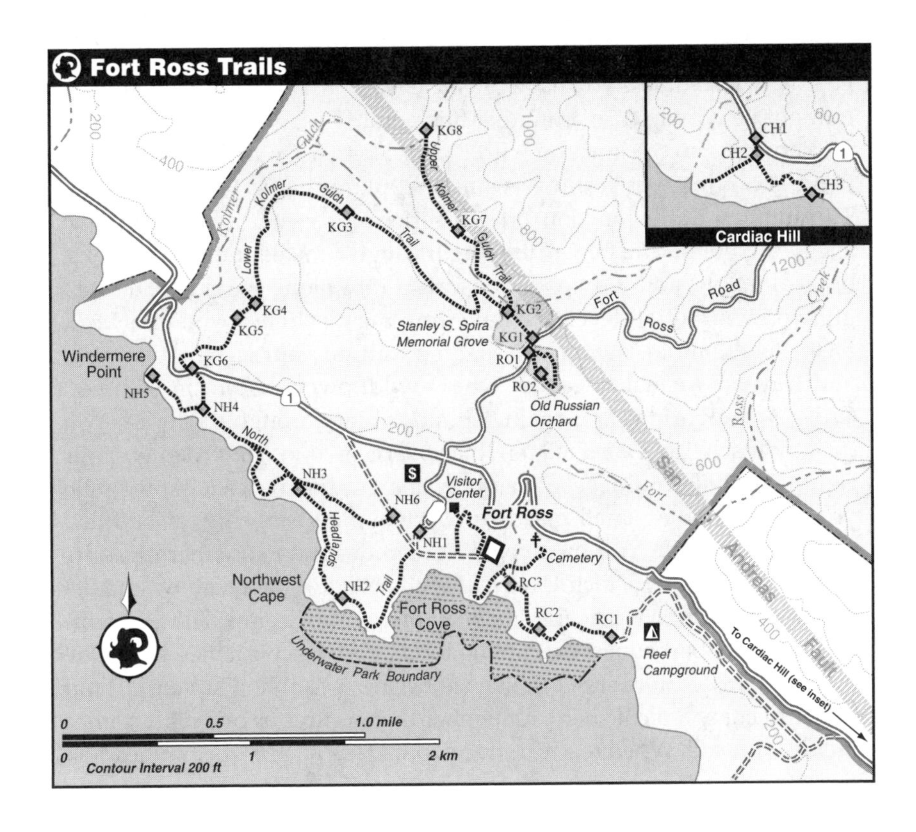

The trail ascends gradually, until at 0.8 mile it begins to level. At 0.9 mile you reach a small meadow. You are well away from traffic noise here, so you may want to settle in for a while and listen to the sounds of the forest. At 1 mile, the trail curves left and begins descending. The light, sandy soil is evidence of the pulverizing effect of the San Andreas Fault on the rock below. The descent increases at 1.3 miles, and at 1.5 miles you duck under a fallen tree. Just beyond, the trail forks. The right fork, an old logging road, descends into Kolmer Gulch. Since it was constructed to help remove logs rather than encourage hikers, it is not maintained now, so take the left fork, a single-track trail you might not initially notice.

At 1.6 miles you reach another small meadow. The ocean soon becomes visible through the forest ahead. At 1.8 miles you break out of the forest into open grassland. The trail veers right, toward a rock outcrop at 1.9 miles. In the distance to the north, you can see the famous Bufano peace statue towering over Timber Cove Inn.

The trail becomes steeper as it descends to a small dirt pullout across Highway 1, so unless you have a vehicle waiting for you at the highway, it might be wise to turn around at this point.

Returning to the junction with Upper Kolmer Gulch Trail, if the sag pond is not too wet you may want to explore this section of the trail. Turning east at the junction, cross a series of plywood planks over the soggy sag pond. You begin climbing through a mixed forest of tanoaks, big-leaf maple, and redwood. The trail climbs along the side of a steep gully on your left. It levels 0.2 mile from the junction as you pass Steer Field Road, an old, overgrown logging trail on your right. At 0.3 mile you traverse a small meadow where wildflowers bloom in summer. Cross a plank bridge and again begin climbing through the forest. You quickly reach Tan Oak Trail, another overgrown logging road on your right. The main trail levels, then begins a gradual descent. At 0.6 mile you reach another small meadow overlooking a stagnant, algae-filled pond on your left. You then begin a steep descent to another meadow at 0.7 mile. Kolmer Gulch Camp, at the far end of the meadow and 0.8 mile from the junction, is the site of an old logging camp. The Call family used it for barbeques. Crumbling remnants of picnic tables, barbeque pits, and an old fort stand in silence beside a babbling stream. If you linger to enjoy a picnic here, remember that no fires or overnight camping are allowed. When ready, retrace your steps back to the trailhead on Fort Ross Road.

Trail 12: Kolmer Gulch Trail Waypoints (WGS84 Datum)

Name	Latitude	Longitude	Feature
KG1	N38° 31.435′	W123° 14.462′	Kolmer Gulch trailhead at Fort Ross Road
KG2	N38° 31.510′	W123° 14.549′	Junction of Upper and Lower Kolmer Gulch Trails
KG3	N38° 31.783′	W123° 15.133′	Small meadow good for a picnic
KG4	N38° 31.532′	W123° 15.462′	Trail junction. Keep left.
KG5	N38° 31.502′	W123° 15.536′	Small meadow.
KG6	N38° 31.349′	W123° 15.692′	Kolmer Gulch trailhead at Highway 1.
KG7	N38° 31.733′	W123° 14.729′	Junction of Upper Kolmer Gulch and Tanoak Trails
KG8	N38° 32.005′	W123° 14.843′	Kolmer Gulch Camp.

Trail 13: North Headlands Trail

Length: 3 miles round trip to Kolmer Beach overlook and Highway 1, 2 hours

Difficulty: Moderate

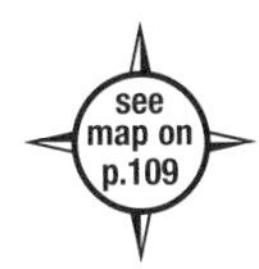

Overview: Although there are no designated trails north of the stockade, a path of sorts traverses the headlands from Northwest Cape to Highway 1 near Windermere Point. The open, windswept headlands offer excellent views of the fort and coastline. You may have to navigate around idly grazing cattle during the hike, for the Parks Department leases this land to local ranchers.

Directions to Trailhead: Take Highway 1 to the Fort Ross main entrance road. Turn west into the park, pay the entrance fee, and park at the west end of the lot.

Trail Description. The trail starts from the southwest end of the main parking lot, where a dirt road departs for the fort. After a short distance the road curves left to join the old route of Highway 1. The old highway also extends to your right, but continue on toward the fort. Just before the speed limit sign is a single-track trail on your right heading toward a fence. Follow this trail through a hiker's gate in the fence at 0.1 mile, then up a saddle through a rocky outcrop. You see various paths departing in either direction. You're welcome to explore any of them, but the described route continues southwest across open grassland toward the cape.

The trail becomes hard to follow, but it really doesn't matter because you have an unobstructed view over the entire route. Study the path shown on the map on Page 109, in general staying near the edge of the bluffs without getting close enough to fall off. You have excellent views of the fort and cove as you head toward the cape.

At 0.3 mile you reach a forest of waist-high yellow bush lupine, with sticky monkeyflower and coast buckwheat growing along the bluff rims. Continue on around the cape, turning northward. The path follows the border between the lupine forest and sandstone outcrops along the ocean.

You exit the lupine forest at 0.7 mile and continue across barren, windswept headlands. At 0.9 mile you reach a 10-foot-deep gulley. The trail turns inland to a crossing point, then back toward the ocean.

You come to an old concrete stock tank at 1.1 miles. The ground here can be muddy all year, so turn inland to find a dry crossing point.

Turning back toward the ocean, you cross several additional gullies and seasonal streams from 1.4 to 1.6 miles. There are several steep volunteer trails to the beach along this section, but they are dangerous and not worth the risk.

At 1.7 miles you reach the intersection with a trail to your right that heads up to a small dirt parking area along Highway 1. (The west trailhead for Lower Kolmer Gulch Trail lies across the highway from this parking area.) Keep left at this intersection, continuing along the headlands trail to its end at 1.9 miles, where you overlook Kolmer Gulch Beach. There is no safe access to the beach from this trail, so you will have to admire it from the bluffs.

For the return trip, retrace your steps or head straight southeast along a dirt road, reaching the old highway at 2.9 miles and the parking lot at just over 3 miles. This shortcut shaves nearly a mile off the total hike.

Trail 13: North Headlands Trail Waypoints (WGS84 Datum)

Name	Latitude	Longitude	Feature
NH1	N38° 30.912′	W123° 14.852′	Trailhead
NH2	N38° 30.722′	W123° 15.177′	Dept of Beaches Survey Benchmark, 1963
NH3	N38° 31.022′	W123° 15.323′	Old concrete stock tank
NH4	N38° 31.246′	W123° 15.666′	Junction with trail to Highway 1
NH5	N38° 31.347′	W123° 15.864′	Kolmer Beach overlook
NH6	N38° 30.942′	W123° 14.975′	Trail junction with old Highway 1

Trail 14: Reef Campground to Fort Ross Cove

Length: 2 miles round trip to Fort Ross Cove

Difficulty: Easy, except for moderate climb near the beginning. The trail passes close to the edge of the bluffs, so watch small children closely.

Overview: This easy trail leads from the northern day-use area to the bluff overlooking Sandy Cove and from there, on to the beach.

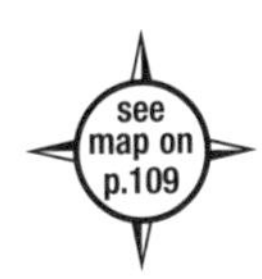

Directions to Trailhead: Take Highway 1 and turn into the Reef Campground entrance at milepost 31.37. Drive to the kiosk, pay the day-use fee, and continue north to the parking area past the campground. Park in the day-use parking lot.

Trail Description. The trail departs from the northwest end of the parking lot. Almost immediately you come to a junction. A short trail to your left ends overlooking the ocean. Take the right fork, which climbs up the side of the bluff. You reach the crest at 0.1 mile, where you look out over the headlands to see the fort a half mile away. The view here looks very much as it would have appeared during the Russian period.

The level but somewhat vague trail then follows the cliff line, where such wildflowers as purple bush lupine, Indian paintbrush, and cow parsnip bloom in spring. At 0.3 mile, you reach another fork. The left path leads to the cove overlook, where you can look down on the beach and imagine what it must have been like in Russian times, when it was bustling with industrial activity. From here, you may be tempted to hike down a steep, narrow path to the beach. Don't do it, as a fall here would result in serious injury or even death. Instead, return to the trail fork and take the right path. This trail winds through the headlands where it eventually descends to the cove at 1.0 mile. After exploring the sandy beach, you can either return the way you came or cross the mouth of Fort Ross Creek and climb the opposite bluff over to the fort.

Trail 14: Reef Campground Trail Waypoints (WGS84 Datum)

Name	Latitude	Longitude	Feature
RC1	N38° 30.602′	W123° 14.185′	Reef Campground trailhead
RC2	N38° 30.623′	W123° 14.445′	Junction with side trail overlooking Sandy Cove
RC3	N38° 30.747′	W123° 14.561′	Sandy Cove trailhead

Trail 15: Orchard Trail

Length: 0.4 mile round trip, 40 minutes

Difficulty: Easy

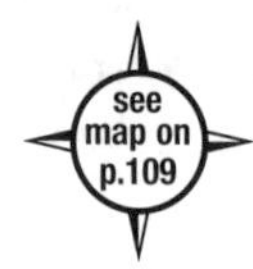

Overview: This easy hike takes you through the old Russian orchard, where several trees planted by the Russians, along with many more planted by later landowners, still survive. Much of the trail traverses open grassland, so use insect repellent to deter ticks and dress appropriately. You may also want to stop first at the visitor center to get the latest information and pick up a map of the orchard, which also includes explanations for the various markers installed throughout the orchard.

Directions to Trailhead: Same as Trail 12, Kolmer Gulch Trail. Rather than parking next to the metal gate at the Kolmer Gulch trailhead, park at the next pullout to the west.

Trail Description: Before starting the hike, take a look at the enormous bay tree just north of the pullout. This ancient giant is hundreds of years old, with a gnarled trunk over 10 feet in diameter. When you're done, cross Fort Ross Road and walk 50 feet south to a wooden gate. Carefully slide it open far enough to get through. Just beyond is a chain link fence with another gate. Carefully unhook the two clasps and this gate flops open slightly. You will probably have to slide it a bit further open to get in. Be sure to close both gates behind you to prevent animals from getting in and damaging the orchard.

A signboard near the gate has a map of the orchard and the locations of the various trees. This is the same map as on the flyer available at the visitor center.

The vague trail heads southeast past apple and pear trees on the right. Volunteers planted the smaller apple trees you see here from cuttings of the original Russian trees in the 1980s. The trail through the orchard is not heavily traveled, so at times you may need to blaze a path through knee-high grass. If in doubt, study the map to get a general idea of where to head.

In 250 feet a short side trail on your right leads to a well-weathered picnic bench. Your trail continues south past wild plums and bitter cherries. At 0.1 mile you have an excellent view of the fort far below. Keep following the vague path southwest toward a stand of redwoods at the orchard's southern fence line. Along the way you pass several olive trees on the left that are possibly from the Russian era.

At 0.2 mile you reach the southern tip of the orchard where several old pear trees still bear fruit. The trail curves sharply left and heads back north through more apple trees. You pass by the olive trees you saw earlier, then head northeast toward a stand of redwoods along the eastern fence line. A redwood here has grown to completely engulf an old pear tree.

Just beyond the redwoods is a broad paddy of horsetail ferns lined by wild blackberry vines. The visitor center map shows the trail passing to the right of the redwoods and through the ferns, but you should keep to the left of the redwoods as you head northeast toward the fence.

The trail passes beside several nice pioneer rose bushes, then curves left and enters a forest of redwoods and apple trees. On your left is a sag pond, an indication you are hiking along the San Andreas Fault. You exit the forest at 0.3 mile, where your trail turns left and crosses the sag pond. After rains, this can be a wet crossing. Scramble up the west bank of the sag pond to its top and then return to the trailhead, visible in the distance at 0.4 mile. Be sure to close both gates when you exit the orchard.

Trail 15: Orchard Trail Waypoints (WGS84 Datum)

Name	Latitude	Longitude	Feature
OR1	N38°31.400′	W123°14.473′	Orchard Trail trailhead
OR2	N38°31.321′	W123°14.428′	View of Fort Ross stockade.

Trail 16: Cardiac Hill

Length: 1.3 miles round trip to beach, 1 hr

Difficulty: Easy to edge of bluffs, strenuous to beach.

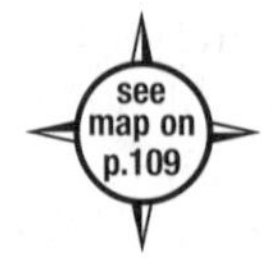

Overview: This trail has two parts. The first is an easy walk across the bluffs to grand views of the coast. Then at the edge of the bluff is a steep, challenging trail down to an isolated, rocky beach 200 feet below. This is a favorite spot for adventurous divers during abalone season. As its name implies, this is not a trail for the casual hiker. In recent years rangers have had to rescue several people who became exhausted or fell and suffered injuries on the climb. Don't attempt this descent unless you are in excellent physical condition and are wearing good hiking boots. A sturdy hiking staff may come in handy as you descend the steepest parts of the trail.

Directions to Trailhead: From Jenner, take Highway 1 north toward Fort Ross. After about 4 miles, watch for the entrance to Vista Trail on the left followed by Meyer's Grade Road on the right. The parking area for Cardiac Hill is a large unmarked dirt pullout on the left, 4.1 miles past Meyer's Grade Road.

Trail Description. The trail starts at the iron gate at the south end of the dirt pullout. Go through the hiker's gate and follow an old ranch road through open grassland. In 250 feet you reach a Y-junction. Take the right fork and follow the old road. In the spring, the wildflowers you may see along here include checkerbloom, blue-eyed grass, scarlet pimpernel, Douglas iris, and suncups.

At 0.1 mile the descent steepens. You have a panoramic view from the bluffs of Fort Ross on the north all the way to Bodega Head on the south. On a clear day you may even see past Bodega Head to Point Reyes far beyond.

You approach the edge of the bluff and the end of the road at 0.3 mile. Although a faint trail leads down to the beach here, it is dangerous and not recommended. Instead, return back to the Y-junction at 0.5 mile and turn right, following the other dirt road south to its end at 0.6 mile. If you aren't prepared for a steep descent, now is the time to turn back.

If you are in good physical condition and are properly equipped, continue down the side of the cliff on a narrow, single-track trail overgrown with coyote brush and purple bush lupine. Look for yarrow, sticky monkeyflower, thimbleberry, horsetail ferns, and poison oak along this part of the trail.

At 0.7 mile the steep trail becomes slippery as you descend through a blue-green clay formation. For this part of the descent you may need to scramble down on your hands and knees. If you have brought along a hiking staff, use it here to maintain your balance.

The slippery clay indicates that you are now traversing the pulverized rock of the San Andreas Fault. This stretch of cliff regularly slides into the sea. Look to the highway far above and observe the massive road reconstruction that was necessary after recent slides.

You reach the rough, rocky beach at 0.8 mile. If you plan to do much exploring, be sure to note the trailhead or mark it as a GPS waypoint, as it may not be obvious when you are ready to return. Explore the beach, including a driftwood fort used by abalone divers a few hundred feet to the south. You'll also see a massive forest of bull kelp floating in the water offshore and various strands that have washed up onto the beach. When ready, return to the trailhead and begin the steep climb back up to the bluff top. Follow the dirt road back to your car for a total distance of 1.3 miles.

Trail 16: Cardiac Hill Waypoints (WGS84 Datum)

Name	Latitude	Longitude	Feature
CH1	38°30.104′ N	W123°13.138′	Cardiac Hill trailhead and parking area
CH2	38°30.057′ N	W123°13.125′	Trail junction
CH3	38°29.945′ N	W123°12.945′	Trailhead at beach

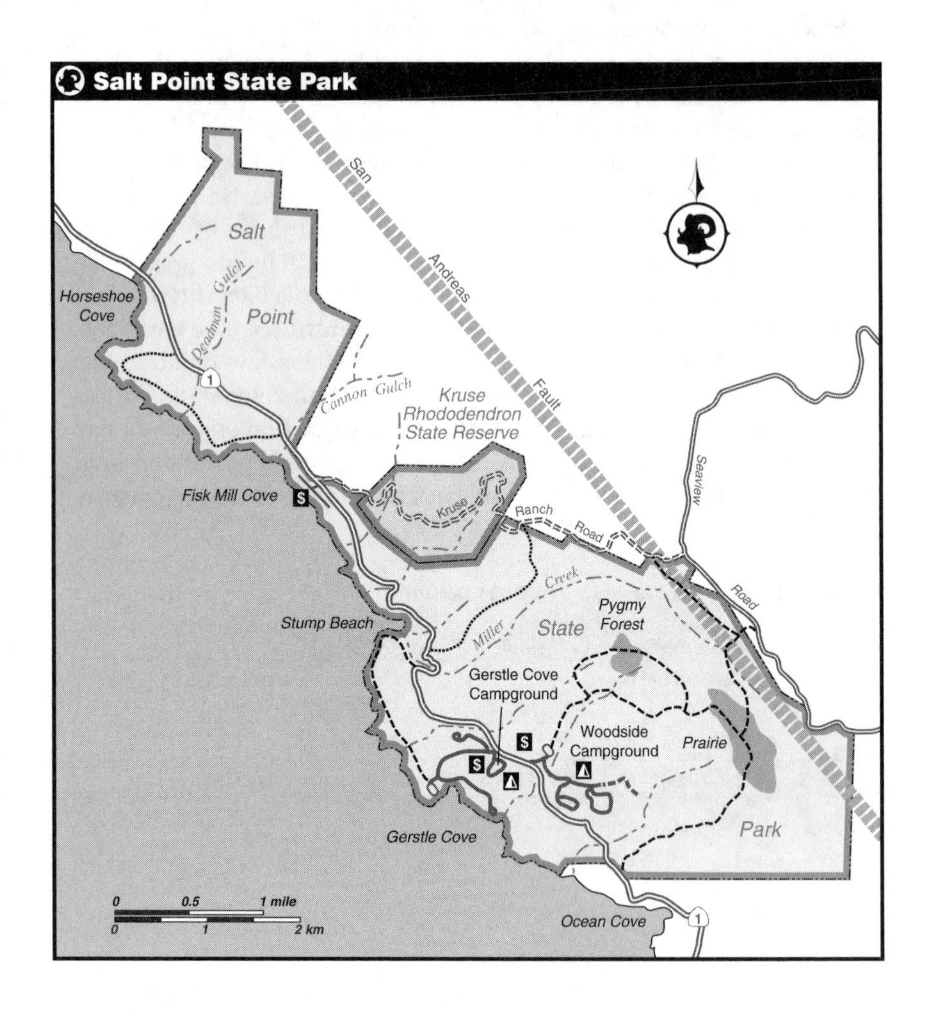
Salt Point State Park
Salt
Point
Horseshoe Cove
Deadman Gulch
Cannon Gulch
San Andreas Fault
Kruse Rhododendron State Reserve
Fisk Mill Cove
Kruse Ranch Road
Seaview Road
Miller Creek
Stump Beach
State
Pygmy Forest
Gerstle Cove Campground
Woodside Campground
Prairie
Park
Gerstle Cove
Ocean Cove
0 0.5 1 mile
0 1 2 km

Chapter 4

Salt Point State Park

The scenic beauty of the Sonoma coast is nowhere more evident than at Salt Point State Park. Here, you'll find rugged cliffs with dramatic ocean views. You'll also see magnificent natural sandstone sculptures, products of the relentless action of wind and waves. On the hills behind the sea you'll walk through quiet forests and grassy meadows, while at the top of the coastal ridge, you'll discover a rare pygmy forest of stunted cypress, pine, and redwood. Twenty miles of trails let you explore the varied terrain and plant communities within the park. Many trails are open to horses, and, from April through October, to well-conditioned mountain bikers as well.

Salt Point's attractions do not stop at the shoreline. It is a favorite destination for abalone divers, who are the leading users of the park. Divers are also drawn to Gerstle Cove Underwater Reserve, one of the first underwater parks in California. Even if you are not a diver you can still experience the wonders of the sea by exploring tidepools at low tide.

Directly adjacent to Salt Point lies Kruse Rhododendron State Natural Reserve. Here, several hiking trails lead through forested canyons where, in the spring, you'll see striking displays of flowering rhododendrons.

Getting There

Salt Point State Park lies along State Highway 1, 20 miles north of Jenner and 8 miles north of Fort Ross. The road is narrow and winding, so figure on at least a 40-minute drive once you leave Jenner. Kruse Rhododendron State Reserve lies along Kruse Ranch Road, a half mile east of its intersection with Highway 1. This is also the way to several trailheads on the east side of Salt Point.

Natural Environment

The park consists of three major environments: coniferous forest, grassland, and brush. Just over three-quarters of the park is covered by forests of coast redwood, Douglas-fir, Bishop pine, tanoak, and madrone. Less than 10 percent is covered in brush, with the remainder consisting of grasslands. The pygmy forest is the result of unusually poor soil conditions in the region of the San Andreas Fault.

In many places, the forest extends right to the ocean. Elsewhere, a buffer of brush and grassland lies between the forest and the sea. Here, you'll find such shrubs as sagebrush, lupine, Indian paintbrush, purple seaside daisy, and cow parsnip, as well as various native perennial and introduced annual grasses. Wildflowers can be spectacular in the spring.

Kruse Rhododendron State Reserve is a mixed forest of tanoak, fir, and second-growth redwood. Many years ago, fire swept through the area, clearing much of the forest and allowing the rhododendrons to flourish. Over time, the forest has started to return—the tanoaks first, followed by Douglas-firs, grand firs, and eventually redwoods. As the conifers take over, the rhododendrons are being squeezed out. The Department of Parks and Recreation thinned out the tanoak trees in the early 1980s as part of their goal of maintaining the beautiful rhododendron displays.

Tafoni. Salt Point is world-renown for its dramatic sandstone formations. A varied assortment of concretions, pedestals, and hollows are the result of 50 million years of wind and water erosion. These elaborate sandstone shapes occur because when the rock originally formed, mineral solutions seeped into the solidifying mass to produce localized

Detail of tafoni sandstone. The intricate structure is probably the result of mineral solutions that seeped along cracks in the dry sand, forming local regions harder than their surroundings.

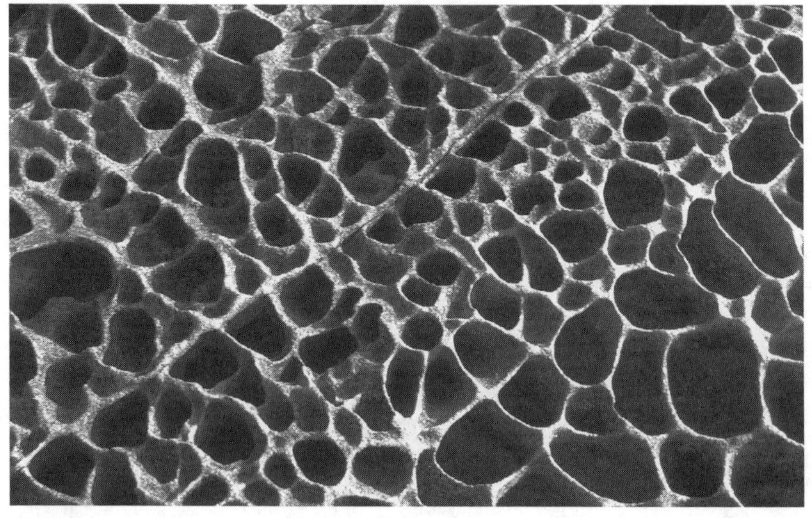

regions harder than the surrounding rock. Once exposed, the softer sandstone eroded away, leaving the harder rock behind. Particularly intriguing are the strange, honeycombed structures known as *tafoni*, a word of Mediterranean origin that has variously been attributed to a Greek word for "tomb" or French and Corsican words for "windows." These waffled shapes were probably formed as the mineral solutions seeped along a series of fractures in the sand comparable to those found on dried mudflats.

Wildlife. Salt Point is home to an abundance of wildlife. Common mammals include the black tailed deer, raccoon, coyote, bobcat, gray fox, striped skunk, badger, squirrel, chipmunk, and field mouse. Wild pigs descended from domestic animals were once common, although concerted efforts to remove them have largely succeeded. And as in much of the west, mountain lions are making a comeback, with several sightings reported each year. Black bear are very rare, with only two recorded sightings over an eight year period. Raccoon and deer are common problems in the campgrounds, so always keep your food protected.

Birds include pelicans, ospreys, and a variety of shore and water-oriented species. You can also watch for gray whales from several spots in the park; Sentinel Rock is an especially good choice.

Abalone Hunting

There seem to be only two opinions of abalone. You either love it or you hate it. Those who love it flock to the Sonoma coast each year to hunt this tasty gastropod. Salt Point is a favorite destination for dedicated divers, but it is also a dangerous area that demands respect. Several people die every year because they overestimate their abilities or underestimate the power of the surf. Before diving, be sure to check the current ocean and dive conditions at www.saltpointoceanconditions.com. The information is updated each morning around 9 A.M. during the abalone season. Also review the rules of ocean safety on Page 18.

Abalone live from the intertidal zone down to depths of several hundred feet, depending on water temperature. They are often found on rocks and crevices exposed to heavy surf. In Northern California it is illegal to use scuba equipment while collecting; you must free dive. The season runs from April through June, then again from August through November.

To remove an abalone, you must pry it loose with a legal-size abalone iron. You are not allowed to use knives, screwdrivers, or sharp instruments. For red abalone the shell must be at least 7 inches across

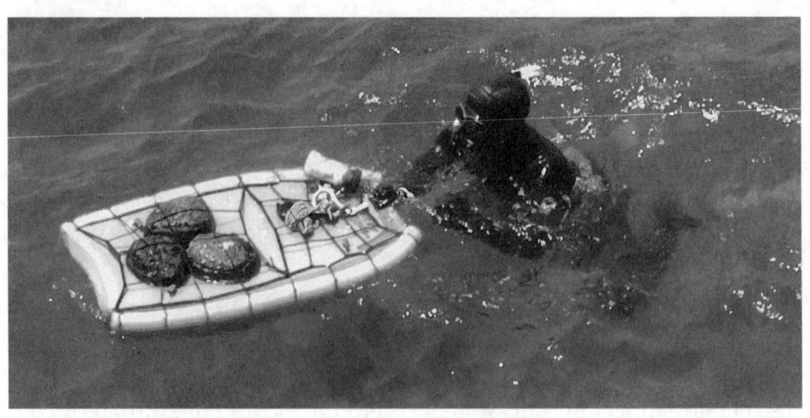
An abalone diver has caught his limit off Fisk Mill Cove.

at its greatest diameter. You can collect a maximum of three abalone per day up to a total of 24 per year. You must immediately return an undersize specimen to the same rock you found it. You must also keep any legal size abalone you detach; you can't exchange a smaller one for a larger one you find later. Abalone must be kept in their shells until you are ready to eat them so game wardens can confirm that your catch meets the minimum size requirement. There are also stringent regulations regarding the use of abalone tags from your Abalone Report Card to mark each catch. For more information refer to the Department of Fish and Game website at www.dfg.ca.gov.

Wardens have stepped up their patrols in recent years because of several well-publicized cases in which tons of abalone were illegally harvested for commercial use. Violators are aggressively prosecuted; heavy fines are routine and prison terms have even been meted out to the worst offenders. Wardens frequently set up inspection checkpoints along Highway 1, so be sure your catch is legal and you have a valid California fishing license in your possession.

Mushroom Collecting

Salt Point is the only state park in the area and one of the few in California presently open to mushroom collecting. You must obtain a permit and pay a nominal fee. For current information, call the Salt Point Ranger Station at 707-847-3221 or the District Headquarters in Duncans Mills, 707-865-2391.

The best time for collecting is in the fall after the first significant rains. You may collect a maximum of 5 pounds per person per day. These must be for your own use and may not be sold. Edible varieties include King and Queen Bolete, various Chanterelles, Coccoli, The Prince, Cauliflower Mushroom, Hedgehog Mushroom, Oyster Mushroom, Candy Caps, Honey Mushroom, Man-on-Horseback, and Shaggy Manes.

The park was closed to collecting during the 1990–91 season because of problems caused by a few insensitive collectors. If it is to remain open in the future, collectors must do their part to minimize the impact of their activities. Observe these important rules:

- Avoid disturbing park vegetation. Try to stay on established trails where possible and do not disturb mushrooms you do not intend to collect.
- Do not rake back the ground cover or dig for mushrooms. An intact ground cover is necessary to ensure continued mushroom fruiting. If you do lift the ground cover to pick a mushroom, remember to place it back down.
- Do not litter. This includes unwanted mushrooms and mushroom trimmings. If you pick a mushroom you do not want, stand it back up to decompose naturally.
- Take only your fair share. Nothing will close the park to collectors faster than people carrying off bucketfuls of mushrooms beyond the legal limit. You are allowed 5 pounds of mushrooms per person per day for your personal use only. You can expect a citation with a stiff fine if you try to take more than this amount.
- Collect only where permitted. Only Salt Point State Park is open to collectors. Collecting is *not* allowed in Kruse Rhododendron State Reserve, Fort Ross State Park, or Stillwater Cove Regional Park. Stay off private land unless you have *written* permission from the landowner to be there.
- Park your car properly. Do not block fire access gates, and pay the day-use fee if you park at Gerstle Cove, Woodside, or Fisk Mill Cove.
- ***Warning!*** There are many poisonous mushrooms in the park. You can die if you eat them. Beginners should always hunt only with an experienced collector. Avoid all mushrooms that even resemble poisonous varieties and be 100 percent certain before eating any of them.

History

The first people to live in the Salt Point region were the Kashaya Pomo Indians. Evidence of their existence can still be found today in the form of refuse piles called *middens*. A midden can be identified because its sterile soil prevents growth of most vegetation. If you come across a midden in your explorations, remember that it is protected by State and Federal law, so leave it undisturbed.

After the Russians left Fort Ross, Mexico began issuing land grants along the northern coast. In 1846, Ernest Rufus and Charles Meyer received the lands stretching from Salt Point to Gualala Point. These two German immigrants called their property, naturally, Rancho German. They owned the land only three years before selling to a partnership

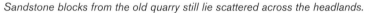

Sandstone blocks from the old quarry still lie scattered across the headlands.

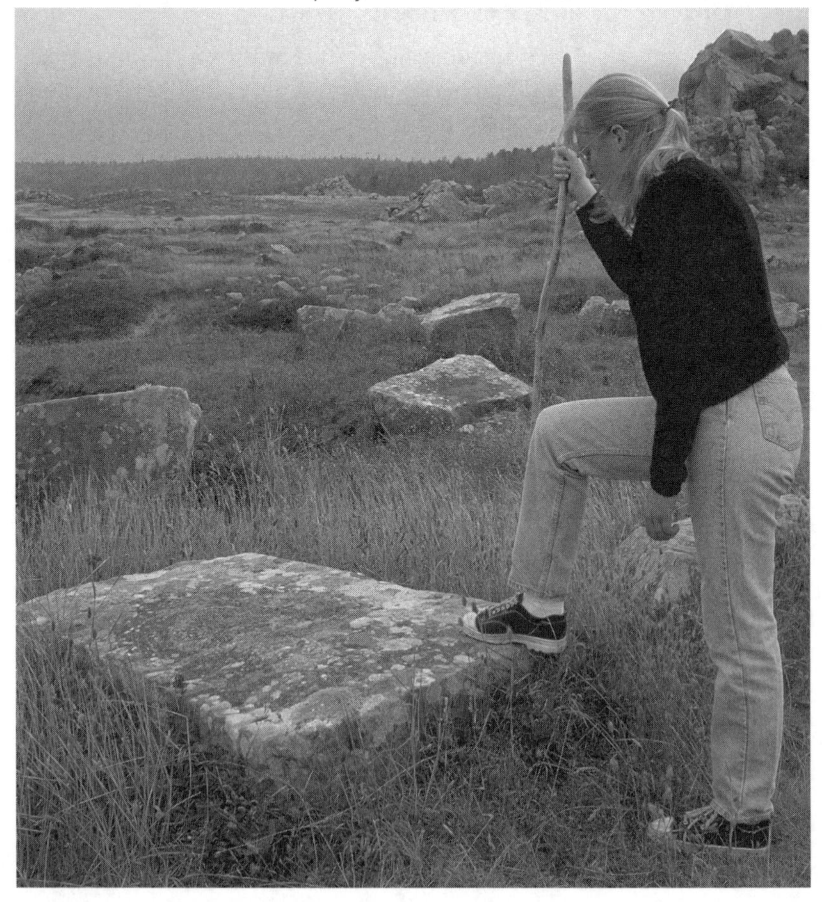

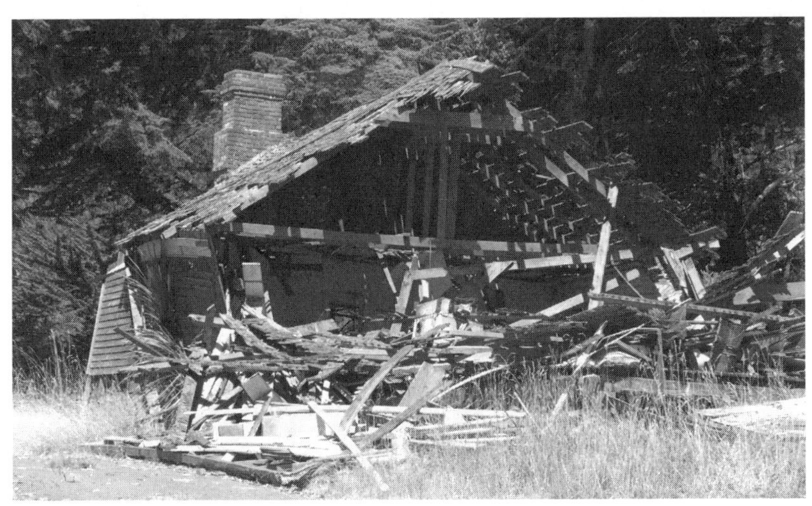

This is all that remains of the 1860s-era post office and Wells Fargo station at Fisk Mill.

that divided it into smaller parcels. Samuel Duncan and Joshua Hendy received the portion that now includes the state park. The two men built a sawmill on the ridge behind Salt Point in 1853. They also leased rights to a San Francisco company to quarry sandstone on their land. Soon, schooners were carrying lumber and stone from Gerstle Cove to the rapidly growing city to the south.

Hendy eventually sold out his interest to Duncan. In 1862, Duncan decided to move his mill south to the present site of Duncan's Landing at Sonoma Coast State Beach. He leased some of his Rancho German land to John Colt Fisk, who settled at Fisk Mill 2 miles north of Salt Point. Fisk built a sawmill, houses, store, hotel, and post office at this site, and a lumber chute for loading schooners at Fisk Mill Cove.

In 1865, Frederick Helmke bought some of Duncan's land, together with Fisk's mill and village. For a time he ran a successful lumber business, but by 1876 the nearby timber had been logged and Helmke moved on.

Duncan sold the remainder of his Rancho German property to Frederick Funcke and Lewis Gerstle in 1870. The two dreamed of forming a prosperous town that would capitalize on San Francisco's booming need for lumber and stone. They founded their town of Louisville overlooking Gerstle Cove in that year and by 1872 had mapped out a plan showing streets all over the headlands. They constructed a number of buildings, including a store, barn, offices, and butcher shop. Their bustling lumber operation included a horse-drawn railway from Salt

Point to Stump Beach. In 1874 they built a two-story hotel, the largest on the Pacific Coast at the time.

Louisville never achieved the grandeur envisioned by its founders. Within 10 years the easily accessible nearby timber had been logged, and the lumber industry fell into decline. Tanbark peeling, an essential source of tannin for hides, remained important, but the region's chief enterprise shifted toward raising sheep and cattle, as it continues today.

Tourism became popular after World War II, with campers and hunters being attracted to the Sonoma Coast area. The State acquired Salt Point in 1968 to provide a recreation facility for the public. Park boundaries have been expanded several times, and campgrounds, trails, and a visitor center have been constructed.

Wildfire of 1993

The park was severely affected by a wildfire started by an illegal campfire in the South Gerstle environmental campground on November 27, 1993. Erratic winds pushed the fire in a northeasterly direction, crossing Highway 1 at various points between Woodside Campground and Stump Beach. The fire was controlled the following day, but not before burning 450 acres and several structures.

You can still see evidence of the fire throughout the park. Dead and blackened trees are evident along the road to the Gerstle Cove day-use area. The environmental campground was destroyed by the fire and will not be reopened. The group campground was also severely damaged, but was reopened five years after the fire.

Fires are a natural part of any forest ecosystem, and they have positive as well as negative effects. At Salt Point, for example, the fire burned away years of accumulated organic matter, exposing the underlying mineral soil. This has helped the germination of many types of plants, most notably Bishop pines and coast redwoods. As you look through the burned areas, you'll see an explosion of young conifers growing in the nutrient-rich soil. Several types of mushrooms also thrive on the burnt ground.

Gerstle Cove Area

The Gerstle Cove area includes a campground, day-use areas, visitor center, marine reserve, and hiking trails. To get there, turn west off Highway 1 at the entrance to Gerstle Cove Campground at milepost

39.90. Pay the entrance fee at the kiosk. The campground is immediately to the left. To reach the visitor center and picnic area, drive down the road 0.5 mile and turn left at the sign. The visitor center is visible on your right 0.2 mile down the road. The picnic area is 0.4 mile past the visitor center. To reach the park's namesake, Salt Point, drive past the visitor center turnoff and continue to the parking lot at the end of the road.

Gerstle Cove Campground

This campground has 30 sites that accommodate trailers up to 27 feet and motor homes to 31 feet. Sites are situated around a tree-lined open meadow. The trees on the ocean side were destroyed in the 1993 wildfire. Sites to the east were spared the worst of the fire.

Each site has a table and fire pit. Restrooms with flush toilets and running water are conveniently located, but there are no showers. Reservations are taken from March 1 through November 30. Call the state park reservation service at 1-800-444-7275. Firewood can be purchased from the camp host near the campground entrance.

A group campground on the north side is available by advance reservation. Check the state parks website at http://parks.ca.gov/for more information.

Visitor Center

The small A-frame visitor center, open weekends 10 A.M.–4 P.M. from April through November (depending on availability of volunteers), directly overlooks the Gerstle Cove Underwater Reserve. Here you can get your questions answered and buy books and postcards related to the park.

Gerstle Cove Picnic Area

This picnic area lies at the end of the road past the visitor center. The pavement ends in a loop with parking spaces at the south side of Gerstle Cove. Just before reaching the loop, you'll see a large pull-out on your right with several picnic tables. Well-maintained cinderblock outhouses sit between the tables and the loop.

Several short trails branch out from the picnic area across the headlands. An easy trail northwest leads 0.4 mile to overlook the underwater reserve. Another trail leads northeast up the ridge to Highway 1 and Woodside Campground. A third trail, starting at a locked gate at the southeast corner of the loop, is not indicated on the official park map. It was once the departure point for the now-closed environmental camp.

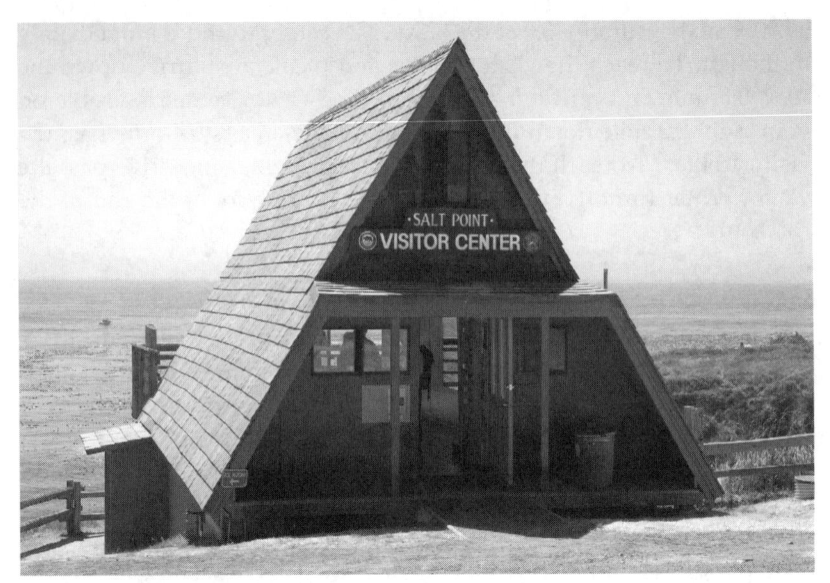

Salt Point Visitor Center.

It extends just over a half mile to the park's southern boundary. Soon after passing the gate, you'll see a steep volunteer trail on your right winding down Squaw Creek to the rocky beach. This access is used by abalone divers to enter the cove.

The rocky point on Gerstle Cove's south end marks the site of the wreck of the steamship *Norlina*, which grounded and sank in a heavy fog the night of August 4, 1926. Rangers assure me the bow is still visible at low tide if you know where to look, though I have never spotted it. The ship's boilers are said to be obvious to divers.

Salt Point Day-Use Area

Salt Point was the spot chosen by Frederick Funcke and Lewis Gerstle for their town of Louisville in 1870. Today, the only evidence of this failed venture lies in the scattered sandstone blocks left over from the stone quarry. A large parking area here gives you access to the headlands and the Gerstle Cove Underwater Reserve. This lot includes a cinderblock restroom structure with a fish-cleaning area and outside showers for divers. A road from the parking area leads down almost to the beach, allowing scuba divers and snorkelers to unload and launch small boats into the cove by hand. You must return your car to the parking lot immediately after unloading your equipment.

A paved, wheelchair-accessible path leads southwest from the parking area, giving you great views of Gerstle Cove and the southern coast. After a few hundred feet the pavement ends but a dirt trail continues on around to the northwestern end of the parking lot to connect with Trail 17. In the late 1800s, this area was the location of a loading chute for schooners anchored in Gerstle Cove. Lumber and sandstone blocks were shipped from here to the city of San Francisco.

Underwater Reserve

The inlet at the north end of Gerstle Cove has been set aside as a reserve within which all marine life is protected. This is an excellent spot to explore the wonders of undersea life. If you intend to dive, be sure you are properly equipped with a wetsuit and float, and follow the rules of dive safety listed on page 19. Abalone divers can swim through the reserve so long as they stay on the surface until well outside its boundaries, marked by bright yellow stripes painted on the rocks at each side of the inlet.

You access the underwater reserve from the Salt Point day-use area. If you have a small boat or kayak, you can drive the paved road almost all the way down to the beach, unload your boat, and return your car to the parking lot above.

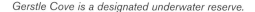

Gerstle Cove is a designated underwater reserve.

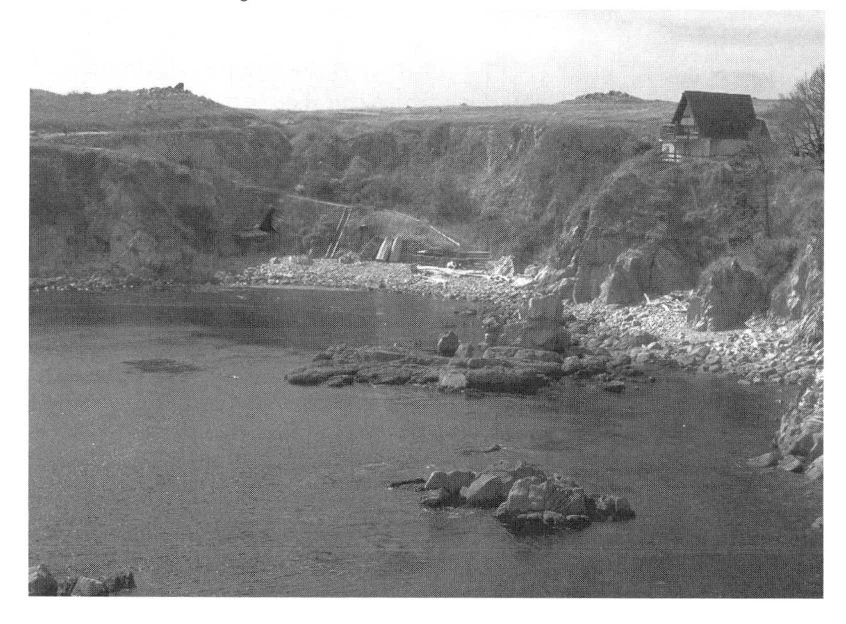

Gerstle Cove is a good place to observe the immense bull kelp forests that grow off Northern California shores. Strands of this massive kelp grow up from deep below the surface, reaching lengths in excess of 100 feet. Each strand ends in a large hollow bulb as much as 6 inches in diameter from which a large number of blades 10–12 feet long hang down. You can often find numerous strands washed onto the shore, especially after a storm.

Woodside Area

The Woodside area, with its campground and hiking trails, lies across Highway 1 from Gerstle Cove. From Highway 1, turn east at the entrance road just south of milepost 39.84 and pay the entrance fee at the kiosk. A modular building on the left serves as park headquarters.

Woodside Campground

The Woodside Campground offers several types of camping experiences. The regular campground consists of 79 sites on two loop roads set in a mixed pine/redwood forest. Restrooms with flush toilets and running water (no showers) are conveniently located, and several sites are disabled accessible. Sites are reasonably secluded, and each has a table and fire ring. Campsites are subject to reservation from March 1 through November 30 by calling the state park reservation service at 1-800-444-7275.

A 20-site walk-in campground provides a more private setting for those who want to fully experience the natural environment. Sites are a half-mile walk from the parking area, and you must carry your equipment to your site. A restroom with running water is located nearby. This campground is on the reservation system from April 1 through November 30, and is open weather permitting. No pets are allowed at this campground.

A hiker/biker campground contains 10 sites reserved for individuals without automobiles. Most users are bicyclists on multi-day rides along Highway 1, but occasionally an adventurous backpacker passes through. These sites are not on the reservation system.

Several well-marked trails branch out from Woodside Campground to the shore at the Gerstle Cove Picnic Area. Another trail parallels the highway from the entrance station southwest to the South Trail trailhead. The most interesting hike is Central Trail, which climbs a wooded ridge to the pygmy forest and prairie (see Trail 18 for a description of this hike).

Northern Areas

Stump Beach

The only sandy beach in the park is located at Stump Beach, and what a beach it is! A sheltered cove with bright white sand and aquamarine water reminds you of a tropical inlet (a comparison you'll soon forget when you feel the cold California water). The sheltering effect of the horseshoe-shaped cove surrounded by high bluffs isolates you from the rough seas, making this a great place for families.

The parking lot, with picnic tables and outhouses, is just off the highway at milepost 41.20. A gravel trail, moderately steep, descends 120 feet to the beach. The fine white sand is covered with the detritus so common to Northern California beaches: bits of driftwood, bull kelp, and an occasional mussel shell. Miller Creek empties on the south side of the beach.

Fisk Mill Cove

This popular day-use site has two picnic areas with a number of tables. It is directly off Highway 1 at milepost 42.63. Be sure to pay the entrance fee when you arrive. The receipt will allow you access into all State Park day-use areas for that day.

The northern picnic area is divided into two lots with a number of parking spaces, including a center section with drive-through spaces for motor homes and vehicles with trailers. The picnic tables, each with an elevated iron barbeque grille, are nestled in a stand of pines 100 feet above the sea. There is also a dual cinderblock restroom with flush

Stump Beach's protected cove and sandy shores make it an ideal picnic spot.

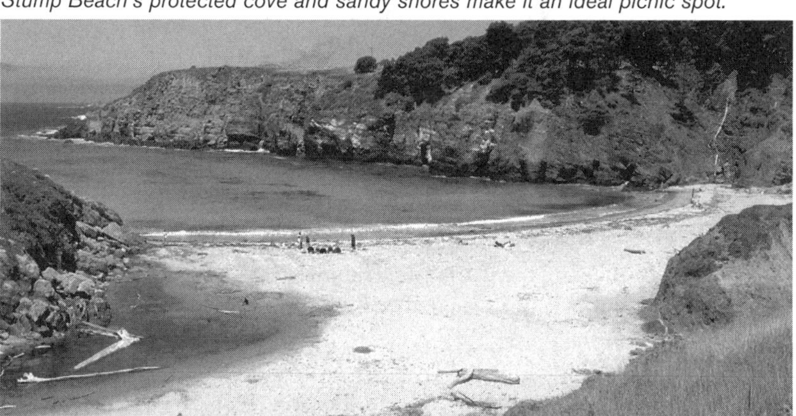

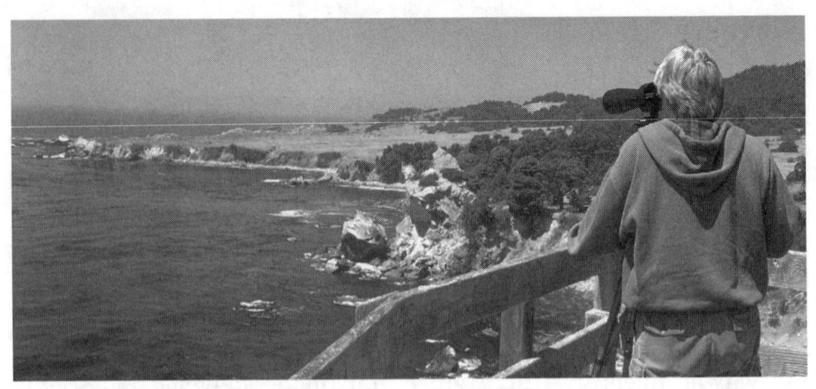

Sentinel Rock is a good spot for seal or whale watching.

toilets. A short path from the center of the first lot connects with Bluff Trail. The path to Sentinel Rock Viewing Platform departs from the end of the second lot.

A smaller parking lot on the south side of the cove ends in a wooded day-use area with picnic tables, elevated barbeque grilles, and a dual cinderblock restroom. Several trails branch out from the picnic area across the bluffs.

Sentinel Rock

A short trail leaves from the northern end of the Fisk Mill Cove picnic area to a viewing platform at Sentinel Rock (refer to Trail 20 for directions.) The viewing platform is a wooden deck at the top of the rock. A bench built into the railing is a good spot to relax and enjoy a picnic lunch. From here, you look out over the coast in all directions. On a clear day, you can see Salt Point to the south and Horseshoe Point to the north. Harbor seals often haul out on the rocks far below, but you'll need a good pair of binoculars to easily observe them.

Kruse Rhododendron State Natural Reserve

Kruse Rhododendron State Natural Reserve was donated to the State in 1933 by Edward P. E. Kruse as a memorial to his father, a founder of San Francisco's German Bank. The area was part of a large ranch established by the family in 1880 on which they raised sheep, harvested tanbark, and conducted logging operations.

This 317-acre park is a living example of how vegetation evolves within a forest. The evolution begins when the original forest is cleared either by fire or by logging operations. In this instance, a severe fire swept through the area many years ago.

The first plants to dominate in the cycle are the fast-growing rhododendrons. For a time, their bright pink blossoms blanket the landscape each spring. Eventually, tanoaks rise up and the rhododendrons begin to decline. The evolution continues as conifers emerge to create a forest of mixed evergreens. Finally, the towering coast redwoods grow to dominate the forest. This complete cycle can take 1,000 years.

Kruse Rhododendron Reserve is now in the tanoak stage with the rhododendrons beginning to decline. The normal philosophy for a state park would be to let nature take its course, but since the park was established for the express purpose of preserving the rhododendron displays, steps have been taken to slow the plant succession. A project to thin the tanoaks was begun in 1979 and completed in 1981. Three years later, significant increases in the floral displays were already evident.

Facilities

The Reserve is a day-use area only, and there are no picnic facilities. Pit toilets are located near the parking lot, a half mile up Kruse Ranch Road. A short loop trail takes you through excellent rhododendron displays before returning to the parking lot. A longer, 2-mile loop gives you a chance to explore the entire park. This rustic trail takes you through mixed forests, shaded canyons, and fine rhododendron displays. In several places, wooden footbridges traverse seasonal streams. The best time to visit is in late April and early May, when the rhododendrons are in full bloom. As a general rule, figure that peak displays occur in the two weeks around Mother's Day.

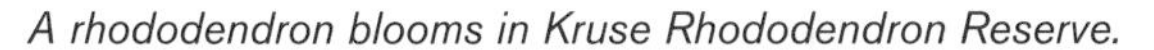
A rhododendron blooms in Kruse Rhododendron Reserve.

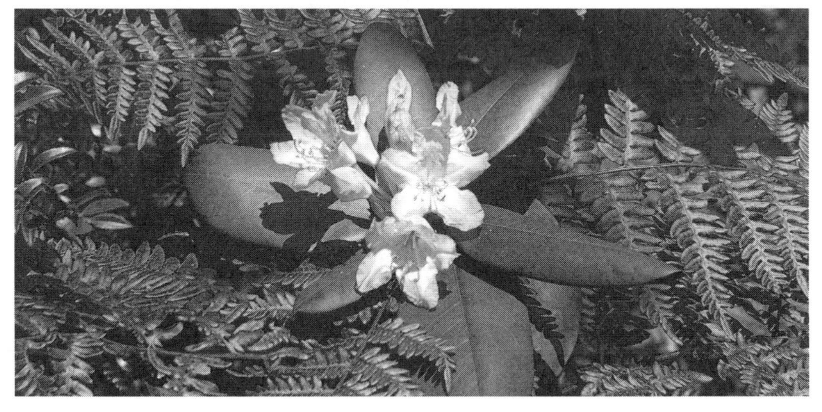

Salt Point State Park Hiking Trails

With over 20 miles of day-use trails, Salt Point State Park offers a variety of hiking experiences. Equestrians and mountain bikers are allowed on any of the broad fire roads, but not on single-track trails. The parks department asks that all visitors stay on developed trails at all times to preserve the natural beauty of the park and to avoid contact with ticks and poison oak.

If magnificent coastal views are your interest, Salt Point Trail, Bluff Trail, and Grace Rock Trail are three good choices. Each follows the edge of the coastal bluffs, where you have excellent views of the surf and the sculpted sandstone features known as tafoni. The exposed headlands can be cold and windy at times, so be sure to bring along a jacket, even in the summer.

For a more challenging hike, take any of the trails up into the hills east of Highway 1. Central Trail out of the Woodside Campground is a good choice. It climbs through mixed forest to the top of the coastal hills, where you'll discover a pygmy forest and grassy prairie. You can also access this trail system from several other points along Highway 1 and from Seaview Road. Be sure to bring snacks and plenty of water for hikes in this area.

The trail through Kruse Rhododendron Reserve is especially popular when the rhododendrons bloom in the month of May. It is a nice hike through shaded redwood forest at any time of the year, so don't limit your visit to a single month. For most of the year you'll probably have this trail to yourself.

Trail 17: Salt Point Trail

Length: 2.7 miles round trip, 1.5 hours

Difficulty: Moderate

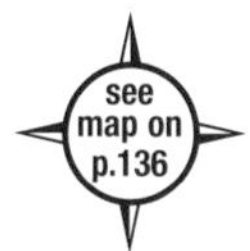

Overview: This relatively level trail north from the Salt Point parking lot to Stump Beach takes you past an old sandstone quarry and the fabled tafoni sandstone outcrops sculpted by wind and wave. As you traverse the headlands you will be treated to spectacular views of the Sonoma coast. As usual when hiking exposed trails along this coast, be prepared for strong winds any time of the year.

Directions to Trailhead: Take Highway 1 to the Gerstle Cove Campground entrance at milepost 39.90 (28 miles north of Bodega Bay). Turn west and pay the entrance fee at the kiosk. Drive past the campground on your left and continue to a parking area all the way at the end of the road, passing the turnoff to the visitor center and picnic area. Park near the trailhead on the northwest end of the lot, away from the restrooms.

Trail Description. The trail starts at an old dirt road that departs from the northwest end of the Salt Point day-use parking lot. In 250 feet the road curves left and another dirt road veers right. Follow the left road for a short distance, then join a single-track trail on your right. Follow this trail northwest toward the shoreline, which you reach at 0.1 mile. Here you will see the first examples of the sculptured, honeycomb-shaped sandstone known as tafoni. You may also see seals lounging on the rocks below.

At 0.2 mile the trail curves right, following the shape of the shoreline around a small cove. You begin to see remains of old sandstone blocks, identified by the lines of drill-holes along their edges, which were quarried to help build the streets of San Francisco over 100 years ago. The large rock outcrop on your right at 0.3 mile was the quarry.

Just past the quarry, you reach an old dirt road. Turn left and follow it northwest for a short distance to a single-track trail on your left. Take this trail and cross Warren Creek, which empties into the cove below. Various trails merge and depart as you continue northwest. Keep to the left, staying close to the shore. You may spot any number of birds as you hike. Especially elegant are the great blue herons that frequent the area. They normally stand in a compact crouch, but when alarmed will extend their necks and bodies straight up to identify the intruder.

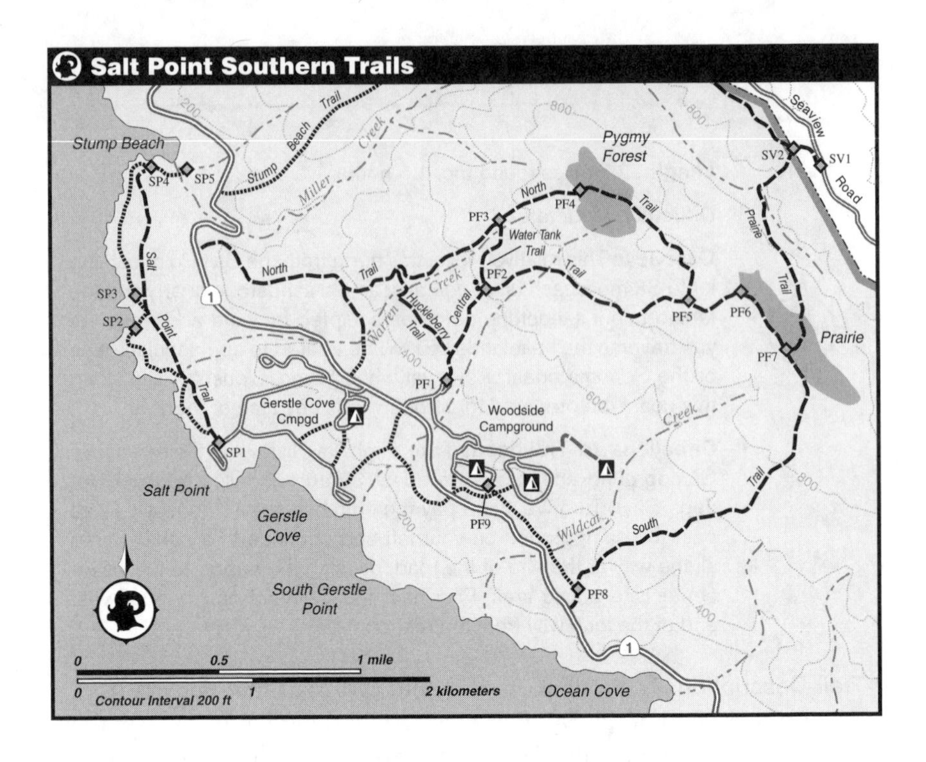

At 0.5 mile a little side trail goes off to rock bluffs on your left. Keep right and rejoin the old road. Follow the road a short distance northwest, then take the single-track trail that veers off on your left.

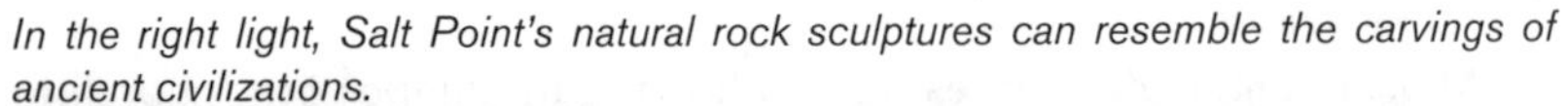

In the right light, Salt Point's natural rock sculptures can resemble the carvings of ancient civilizations.

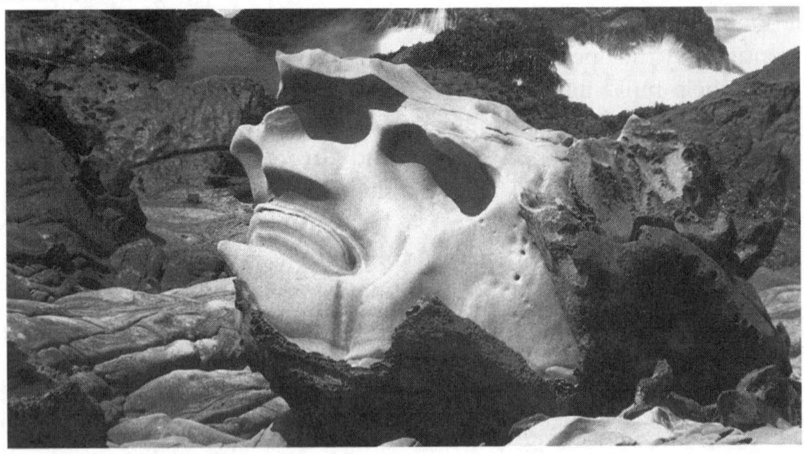

At about 0.9 mile the trail climbs a small saddle between rock outcrops. As you emerge, you see a broad expanse of intricately sculpted sandstone along the shore. You can detour here to explore the fantastic shapes reminiscent of sandstone hoodoos in southern Utah. Stay back from the surf, as the sea is unpredictable. It may appear fairly calm for extended periods, but then be punctuated by an enormous breaker that crashes violently onto the rocks, sending spray 50 feet into the air.

The local Kashaya Pomo Indians once collected salt from this area for their own use and as a trading commodity. The sandstone forms natural catch basins for seawater, and when the water evaporates the salt is left behind. The Kashaya gathered it to trade for goods such as obsidian from inland tribes. It was this early commercial activity that gave Salt Point its name.

You pass through a brushy area with numerous chest-high yellow bush lupines at 1.0 mile. A sandy area on your left leads to more tafoni formations. Also look for numerous sea palms along the shoreline below you.

Carefully cross another seasonal creek at 1.1 miles and keep to the left, staying close to the bluff. The trail curves right at 1.3 miles, following the shape of the shoreline. Stump Beach is visible ahead, far below.

At 1.5 miles the trail descends the bluff to Stump Beach, which has the only sandy beach in the park. When you reach the beach, take careful note of the trailhead, as it may not be obvious when you return. If you have a GPS receiver, mark the trailhead as a waypoint so you can find it easily when you are ready to return.

Unless you have parked a second vehicle at the Stump Beach parking area, you will need to return the way you came. You can cut 0.4 mile off the return trip by staying on the broad dirt road all the way back to the Salt Point trailhead.

Trail 17: Salt Point Trail Waypoints (WGS84 Datum)

Name	Latitude	Longitude	Feature
SP1	N38° 34.041′	W123° 19.983′	Trailhead
SP2	N38° 34.381′	W123° 20.307′	Quarried sandstone rocks with drill marks on edges
SP3	N38° 34.476′	W123° 20.313′	Good tafoni formations
SP4	N38° 34.865′	W123° 20.263′	Trail junction with dirt road
SP5	N38° 34.832′	W123° 20.142′	Trailhead at Stump Beach

Trail 18: Central Trail to Pygmy Forest and Prairie

Length: 4.6 mile loop (1.0 mile to pygmy forest, 1.9 miles to prairie), 2.5 hours. Shorter loops possible.

Difficulty: Strenuous

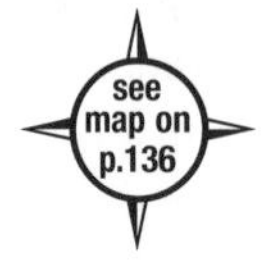

Overview: This trail climbs 600 feet through coastal redwoods to a rare pygmy forest, then on to a "prairie," an area of open grassland high in the hills. Numerous signs along the initial part of the hike introduce you to the many trees, shrubs, and flowers of the forest. You then start a long descent through more redwood forest to Highway 1 and the trailhead. For most of the hike you travel along broad fire roads, but the last mile is on a single-track trail with several short but steep climbs and descents. You aren't likely to encounter many other hikers along most of the route.

Directions to Trailhead: From Highway 1 turn east into Woodside Campground, pay the entrance fee, and drive in. The trailhead lies on your left at the day-use parking lot just behind the park headquarters.

Trail Description. The trail is a well-maintained old logging road that starts from a gate at the north end of the parking lot. You begin a steady, moderately steep climb through mixed forest of pine, fir, tanoak, madrone, and redwood. The understory includes manzanita, rhododendron, redwood sorrel, and trillium. As you climb toward the pygmy forest, look for numerous trailside signs that describe the ferns, trees, and shrubs of the forest.

At 0.1 mile you come to the junction with Huckleberry Trail on your left. It leads to North Trail, your eventual destination, but for now it is better to stay on Central Trail rather than turning left here. Continue to the right on a steady climb with only an occasional brief relief from the ascent. Huckleberries and salal, both with edible black berries in the late summer, line the trail. As you hike through the forest, notice the numerous trees that were blown over by strong storm winds during the winter of 2007–2008.

At 0.4 mile you come to four water tanks on the left that provide water for the park. Turn left here onto Water Tank Trail, another broad fire road leading to North Trail. You finally get a respite from the climb, as this road is fairly level for most of its 0.3-mile length. Look for sword ferns, deer ferns, horsetail ferns, and western chain ferns along the trail.

The junction with North Trail is marked by a stretch of yellow-orange sandy soil. Turn right and resume your steady climb. Tan oaks dominate the forest now; their leaves cover the steep trail, making for a slippery path. As you curve left, then right again, notice a hollow stump on your right, blackened by campfires of years past, with a log bench next to it. Remember that open fires are now illegal—their disastrous results are only too evident in the forest surrounding Gerstle Cove.

The trail levels and the forest thins when you arrive at the pygmy forest after hiking 1.0 mile. Notice the rough, sandy soil that forms only a shallow layer over a bedrock of iron and graywacke sandstone. This region lies over the San Andreas Fault and has been pulverized by eons of geologic activity. Stunted Bishop pines, redwoods, cypress, manzanita, and bay trees struggle to extract nutrients from the poor soil.

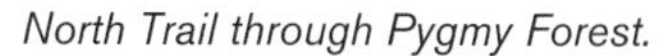
North Trail through Pygmy Forest.

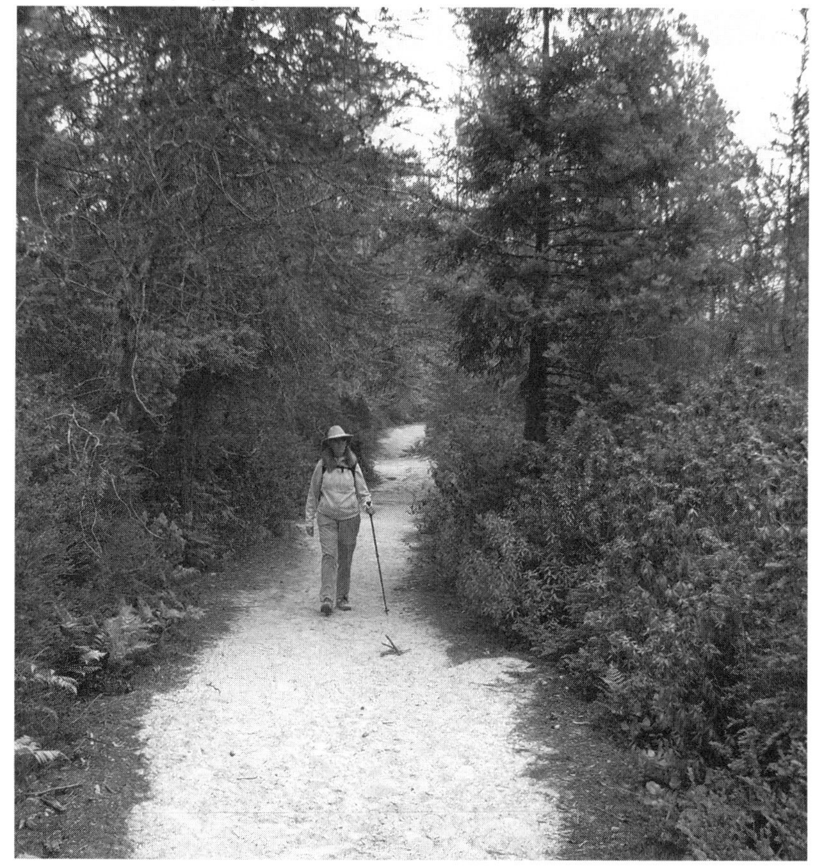

You walk through true pygmy forest for about 0.3 mile. As you transition out, you climb through a Bishop pine forest lined with tanoaks, bracken ferns, huckleberries, salal, and Labrador tea, to reach the highest point of the trail at 900 feet elevation. You then descend back to a junction with Central Trail.

You have several choices at this point. For the shortest hike, turn right and walk down Central Trail, reaching the trailhead after a total hike of 3 miles. Or you can return the way you came for a 3.5-mile hike. If you're still energetic, though, turn left and follow Central Trail through the pine forest to a large open prairie at 1.9 miles. Your trail skirts the west edge of the prairie, with a Monterrey pine forest on your right.

Central Trail ends at a junction at 2.2 miles. On your left is Prairie Trail, which crosses the prairie and climbs steeply to a trailhead at Seaview Road, or over to Kruse Ranch Road via Plantation Trail. Straight ahead is South Trail, which goes back down to Highway 1. Take this route. You soon leave the prairie and reenter a dense forest, beginning a descent at 2.4 miles. Initially, the descent is gradual, but it soon becomes steeper. Large numbers of redwood stumps and fairy rings show that this area was heavily logged long ago.

You reach the bottom of the steepest descent at 2.9 miles and leave the densest forest at 3.3 miles. The junction with Power Line Trail is on your right at 3.5 miles, just before Highway 1. Turn right here and follow a single-track trail through a pine forest that was clear-cut just wide enough for the power lines. Your trail now parallels the highway back to Woodside Campground. Initially, the trail is fairly level, with bunch grass, salal, deer ferns, and bracken ferns along the route. At 3.6 miles you make a steep descent to cross Wildcat Creek, then climb steeply up the other side. In the rainy season, you may have to detour over to nearby Highway 1 to make this crossing.

A trail joins from the left at 3.8 miles. Continue straight ahead to another trail junction at 3.9 miles, just at the outer edge of the campground. Continue straight to immediately reach the paved campground road. Take this road 0.6 mile back to your car at the day-use parking area, for a total hike of 4.6 miles.

Trail 18: Central Trail to Pygmy Forest and Prairie Waypoints (WGS84 Datum)

Name	Latitude	Longitude	Feature
PF1	N38° 34.212′	W123° 19.110′	Central Trail trailhead at Woodside Campground
PF2	N38° 34.496′	W123° 18.941′	Junction of Central Trail and Water Tank Trail
PF3	N38° 34.688′	W123° 18.888′	Junction of Water Tank Trail and North Trail
PF4	N38° 34.791′	W123° 18.559′	Pygmy Forest
PF5	N38° 34.454′	W123° 18.140′	Junction of North Trail and Central Trail
PF6	N38° 34.480′	W123° 17.936′	Enter prairie
PF7	N38° 34.311′	W123° 17.770′	Junction of Central, South, and Prairie Trails
PF8	N38° 33.613′	W123° 18.583′	Junction of South Trail and Powerline Trail
PF9	N38° 33.912′	W123° 18.929′	Junction of Powerline Trail and campground road
SV1	N38° 34.849′	W123° 17.614′	Prairie Trail trailhead at Seaview Road
SV2	N38° 34.906′	W123° 17.717′	Junction of Prairie Trail and Plantation Trail

Trail 19: Bluff Trail from Fisk Mill Cove to Stump Beach

Length: 2.8 miles round trip, 1.5 hours

Difficulty: Moderate

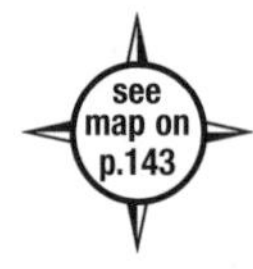

Overview: This trail stretches from the bluffs overlooking Stump Beach all the way to Horseshoe Point, but most people will want to start from either Fisk Mill Cove or nearby Cannon Gulch. This trail description covers the southerly hike from Fisk Mill Cove to Stump Beach. The following description covers the northerly hike to Horseshoe Cove. You can also enter Bluff Trail from the free parking area along Highway 1 just north of Fisk Mill Cove at Cannon Gulch.

Directions to Trailhead: Drive to Fisk Mill Cove, pay the entrance fee, and turn left. Drive all the way to the end of the road and park at the southern day-use picnic area. A short spur trail from here connects with the main trail.

Trail Description. From the parking lot, go west through the picnic area for 200 feet to Bluff Trail. Turn left at this junction and go under a stand of Bishop pines. Your trail follows the bluffs along Fisk Mill Cove, where a massive forest of bull kelp floats for much of the year. Bull kelp is the fastest growing seaweed in the world, adding as much as 10 inches in a single day. It completes its entire life cycle in one year.

The somewhat vague trail continues south through pine forests, bunch grass, and bracken ferns. Watch for poison oak along the way. You emerge from the forest on a bluff overlooking Fisk Mill Cove at 0.1 mile. Go down a series of wooden steps with a railing directly along the edge of the bluff.

At 0.2 mile you come to a junction with a trail on your left that goes up the bluff to the campgrounds. Continue south and go under a large fallen Douglas-fir, then pass beside a rock outcrop on your left with hollows carved by wind and wave. You reach a wooden bridge over Chinese Gulch at 0.3 mile. The trail again becomes a bit vague, so keep right and stay along the edge of the bluff, where you have good views of sandstone outcrops at the waterline below you.

Another trail heads up to the highway at 0.4 mile. Continue south through bush lupine and purple seaside daisies. Two rusted metal poles embedded in rock at 0.6 mile mark a rough trail down to a rocky beach. Continuing on, you reach Phillips Gulch at 0.8 mile. There is no bridge here, so you will have to rock-hop across the running water. As you climb up the other side, the trail splits to go around a sandstone outcrop. Stay to the right, close to the edge of the bluff. You have a great view of Horseshoe Point beyond Stump Beach.

As you climb to the top of a hill at 0.9 mile, you get a good view of Stump Beach ahead on your left. From here, you can easily see why this sheltered, sandy beach at the end of a narrow inlet is fairly calm even on stormy days.

You walk through Bishop pines at 1.0 mile and quickly pass under a telephone line. A telephone pole here lies in the center of a 20-foot circle that has been cleared of vegetation. At the telephone pole, take the trail that goes off to the left toward the road. You pass under two fallen trees at 1.1 miles, then turn east and cross a dry gulch. At 1.3 miles, your trail descends a gulch to the north side of Stump Beach. Cross a creek and arrive at the beach at 1.4 miles. Another trail at this junction heads up to the Stump Beach parking lot. If you have arranged a shuttle, this is the

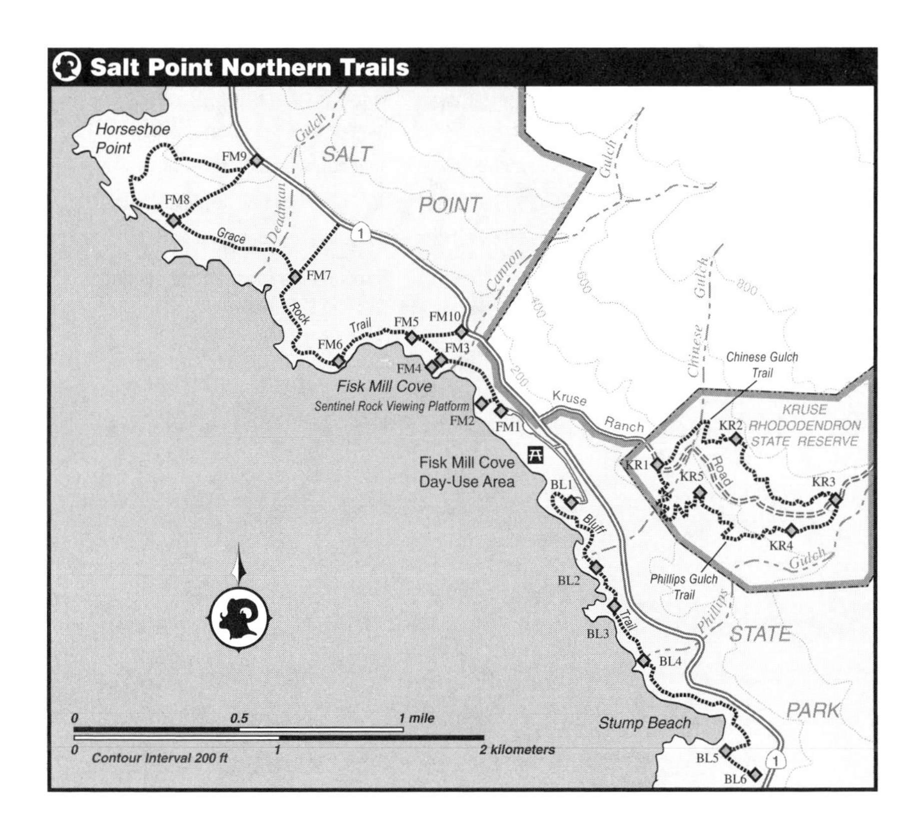

route to take. Otherwise, it's time to turn around and retrace your steps back to Fisk Mill Cove.

Trails 19–20: Bluff Trail, Grace Rock Trail Waypoints (WGS84 Datum)

Name	Latitude	Longitude	Feature
BL1	N38° 35.499′	W123° 20.619′	Bluff Trail trailhead at Fisk Mill Cove
BL2	N38° 35.334′	W123° 20.558′	Junction with trail to highway
BL3	N38° 35.237′	W123° 20.501′	Side trail to bluff overlooking ocean
BL4	N38° 35.100′	W123° 20.405′	Phillips Gulch trail crossing
BL5	N38° 34.860′	W123° 20.107′	Bluff Trail trailhead at Stump Beach
BL6	N38° 34.803′	W123° 20.028′	Stump Beach parking lot
FM1	N38° 35.733′	W123° 20.874′	Grace Rock Trail trailhead at Fisk Mill Cove
FM2	N38° 35.744′	W123° 20.950′	Sentinel Cove Viewing Platform
FM3	N38° 35.867′	W123° 21.086′	Junction with trail to Fisk family cemetery
FM4	N38° 35.853′	W123° 21.104′	Fisk family cemetery
FM5	N38° 35.917′	W123° 21.129′	Junction with trail from Cannon Gulch parking area
FM6	N38° 35.852′	W123° 21.417′	Rusted iron ring from 19th century lumber chute
FM7	N38° 36.076′	W123° 21.574′	Junction with side trail to highway
FM8	N38° 36.217′	W123° 21.984′	Junction with trail to parking area
FM9	N38° 36.371′	W123° 21.705′	Parking area on Highway 1
FM10	N38° 35.931′	W123° 20.992′	Parking area for alternate starting point at Cannon Gulch

Trail 20: Grace Rock Trail from Fisk Mill Cove to Horseshoe Point

Length: 4.3 miles round trip, 2 hours.

Difficulty: Moderate

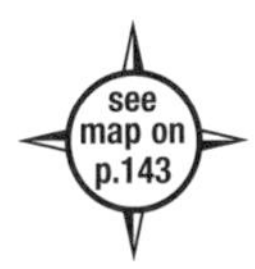

Overview: This trail takes you through the sandstone-sculptured northern half of Bluff Trail, now called Grace Rock Trail on park maps. Along the way you will discover a pioneer cemetery and the remains of an old lumber chute used to load sailing ships in the 19th century. It's also the way to the viewing platform at Sentinel Rock, only a short distance from the trailhead.

Directions to Trailhead: Drive to Fisk Mill Cove, pay the entrance fee, turn right, and park in the most northerly parking lot. The trailhead is at the north end of the parking lot.

Trail Description. From the trailhead, hike north through a forest of Bishop pines and occasional poison oak. In 200 feet, you reach a signed junction indicating that Bluff Trail turns right. Rather than turning here, go straight ahead to another sign pointing to Sentinel Rock on the left. Take this trail up the side of a wooded bluff to the grand views of Sentinel Rock Viewing Platform at 0.1 mile. Be alert for the poison oak that grows profusely along this stretch of trail.

Return back to the Bluff Trail sign at 0.2 mile and turn left along a faint trail through the forest. Bracken ferns line your path along this stretch. You begin a descent into Cannon Gulch at 0.3 mile and reach the bottom at 0.4 mile. If the water isn't running too high, you can step carefully across the gulch, but in the wet season, it may be impassible. If so, you will need to go back and start your hike from the Highway 1 trailhead on the north side of Cannon Gulch.

As you climb out of the gulch, you reach a three-way trail junction near a rock outcrop and adjacent stand of Bishop pines. The trail on the right eventually reaches the Highway 1 trailhead at Cannon Gulch. Bluff Trail continues straight ahead, and the trail on your left goes west to the edge of a cliff. Take this short side trail to the Fisk family cemetery on a peaceful bluff. Among the several graves here is a marble column marking the final resting spot of 42-year-old Andrew Fisk and his 6-month old daughter, Clara Belle, who died within days of each other in 1874. The faded stone inscription reads *"Of such is the kingdom of heaven."*

Return to the three-way junction and take Bluff Trail northeast past a dilapidated wooden outhouse, now well over a century old. You reach a broad dirt road entering from the right at 0.6 mile. This is where you would enter if you had started from the Highway 1 trailhead at Cannon Gulch. Continue northwest on this road and pass through an old fence line to a small, wooded gulch where a steep, dangerous spur trail descends to a rocky beach. Cross the gulch and emerge into grassland where various trails enter and depart. Stay on the main, well-worn path that follows the edge of the headlands.

At 0.8 mile you pass a picnic table on your right and a metal sign describing the history of Fisk Mill Cove. The trail curves left toward a rock outcrop at the north end of the cove. A conspicuous wooden post is visible in the distance. As you bear left of the post, you see several old iron rings embedded in the rock. These and the post are remnants of a lumber chute used to load schooners in the mid 1800s. Veer north past the rock outcrop to see a number of weathered wooden beams from the chute lying on the ground.

As you continue along the coastline, notice the geology of the shore. Soft yellow sandstone is being eroded away, leaving behind darker gray concretions. Stay back from the surf here, for even on relatively calm days an occasional rogue wave will crash dangerously over the rocks.

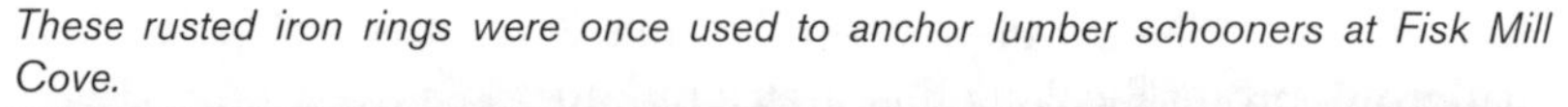
These rusted iron rings were once used to anchor lumber schooners at Fisk Mill Cove.

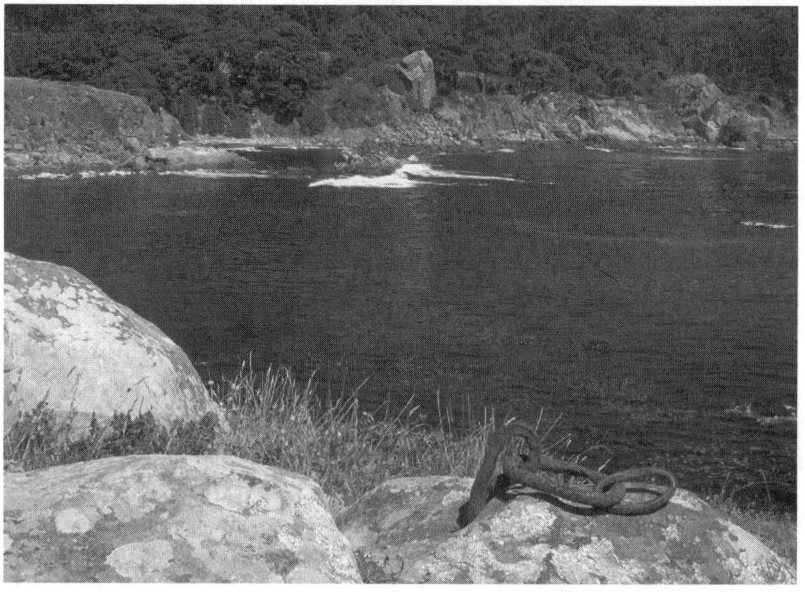

Your trail traverses a low forest of bush lupine at 1.1 miles. In the spring and early summer, the flowers on these shrubs can be a sea of yellow. Pass between two low sandstone outcrops at 1.3 miles and leave the lupine forest.

Numerous volunteer trails enter and depart along this stretch. Follow the broad dirt road generally northwest, reaching a stand of trees and a flowing brook at 1.5 miles. This is Deadman Gulch. There can be running water here even in late summer, so pick your way carefully along the rocks of the gulch. Deadman Gulch should more properly be named *Deadmen* Gulch, for this treacherous stretch of coastline has claimed the life of more than one careless fisherman.

At 1.7 miles you reach a broad trail heading north to the highway. This will be your return path, but for now, continue straight ahead. You pass more sandstone and tafoni at 2.0 miles, just as the road curves right and heads up the hill. From here, you climb steadily through open grassland and an occasional Bishop pine, reaching the highway at milepost 43.66 after having traveled 2.6 miles. For your return trip, take the same trail back for a few hundred feet to a junction. Take the left fork and return to Bluff Trail just west of Deadman Gulch, then go left to retrace your steps. From here, it is another 1.4 miles back to your car, for a total distance of 4.3 miles.

Trail 21: Kruse Rhododendron Loop

Length: 1.9 miles round trip, 1.5 hours

Difficulty: Moderate

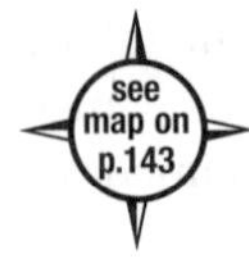

Overview: This is a popular hike when the rhododendrons are in bloom in April and May. At other times of year you are likely to have the trail to yourself. Don't restrict yourself just to rhododendron season–it is a pleasant hike through redwood forest at any time of year. The described hike is an extended loop through the park. If you're just interested in seeing rhododendrons, you can take a much shorter loop through the best displays right near the trailhead.

Directions to Trailhead: Take Highway 1 to the junction with Kruse Ranch Road, just north of the Fisk Mill Cove Day Use Area. Turn east and park in the Kruse Rhododendron parking area a half mile up the road. There are spaces for about 10 cars in parking spots on either side of the road.

Trail Description. The trail begins on the north side of the road, at the stairs on the right side of the parking area. This is the Rhododendron Loop Trail, with dense displays on either side of the trail. A split log rail fence keeps you on the trail and protects the delicate plants. In addition to the rhododendrons, you'll also see huckleberries, tanoaks, bracken ferns, redwoods, and Douglas-firs.

In 300 feet, Rhododendron Loop Trail turns left and quickly goes back to the parking lot. Continue past this junction and on into the forest. You are now making a slow climb along the north side of a ravine on Chinese Gulch Trail. There are numerous redwood stumps and fairy rings along the trail, remnants of when the region was logged in the late 19th and early 20th centuries.

You reach a local summit at 0.2 mile, then descend to a bridge across a creek. Climb steeply up wooden steps on the other side of this gulch to a forest of redwoods, tanoaks, rhododendrons, bracken ferns, sword ferns, and huckleberries. Old log benches at several points along the way provide a chance to sit and enjoy the solitude of the forest.

Your trail, which has been climbing near the road, turns away from it at 0.5 mile. You soon reach a junction. A trail on the right returns down to the road, giving you the opportunity for a shorter hike.

Your climb levels at 0.6 mile and starts descending. Throughout the forest you see evidence of trees that were blown over by strong storm

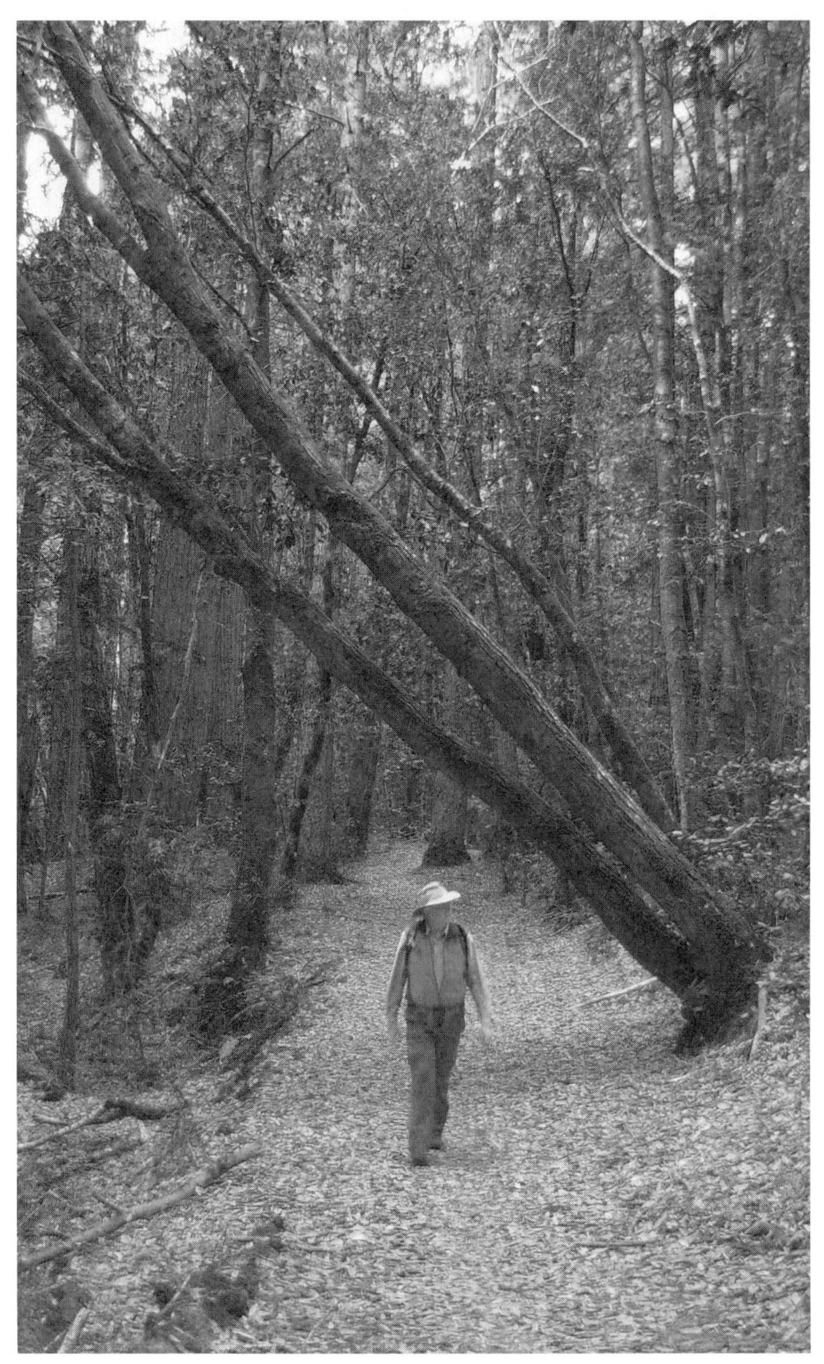

Hiker along Phillips Gulch Trail.

winds in the winter of 2007–2008, including a madrone that has fallen across the path and has not been cleared. It is easy enough to walk around. Cross another wooden bridge across a gulley filled with sword ferns at 0.8 mile. There are more fairy rings along here, including one with a so-called goosepen formed by the burned-out hulk of the central stump. Labrador tea, huckleberries, and wax myrtle grow along the trail.

Step over another fallen log and descend to the road, which you reach at 1.0 mile. When you cross the road, you are now on Phillips Gulch Trail. You descend through a heavy mixed forest of redwoods, firs, bay trees, and tanoaks. Go around a fallen redwood at 1.1 miles and quickly reach a large fairy ring. This is a good example of a second-generation fairy ring. Not only has the central tree fallen, but the secondary sprouts have also fallen. The new trunks are third-generation sprouts.

The trail briefly levels, but after crossing two wooden bridges you resume your descent. You curve right to go around a deep gulley at 1.3 miles. Cross a wooden bridge and pass another example of a multi-generational fairy ring at 1.4 miles. You soon reach a junction where a side trail goes back up to the road. Continue on Phillips Gulch Trail, as the side trail won't save you much time.

At 1.5 miles, you reach the best example of a fairy ring along the trail. This fine, multi-generation ring is almost like a cathedral in the center. Not all fairy rings are the result of logging. This one predates the logging era and is a result of natural causes.

You now begin a steeper descent as you loop back and forth down the east side of Chinese Gulch. At the bottom of your descent, cross a bridge over the creek and begin a steady climb up the other side. You have fine views of the gulch as you climb.

You pass beside a rotting log bench at 1.8 miles and soon see restrooms in the forest on your left. It's now just a short hike back to the parking lot and your car, which you reach at 1.9 miles.

Trail 21: Kruse Rhododendron Loop Trail Waypoints (WGS84 Datum)

Name	Latitude	Longitude	Feature
KR1	N38° 35.575′	W123° 20.352′	Kruse Rhododendron trailhead
KR2	N38° 35.652′	W123° 20.089′	Junction with side trail to Phillips Gulch Trail
KR3	N38° 35.505′	W123° 19.751′	Junction with Kruse Ranch Road
KR4	N38° 35.424′	W123° 19.904′	Nice multi-generation fairy ring
KR5	N38° 35.522′	W123° 20.202′	Junction with side trail to Chinese Gulch Trail

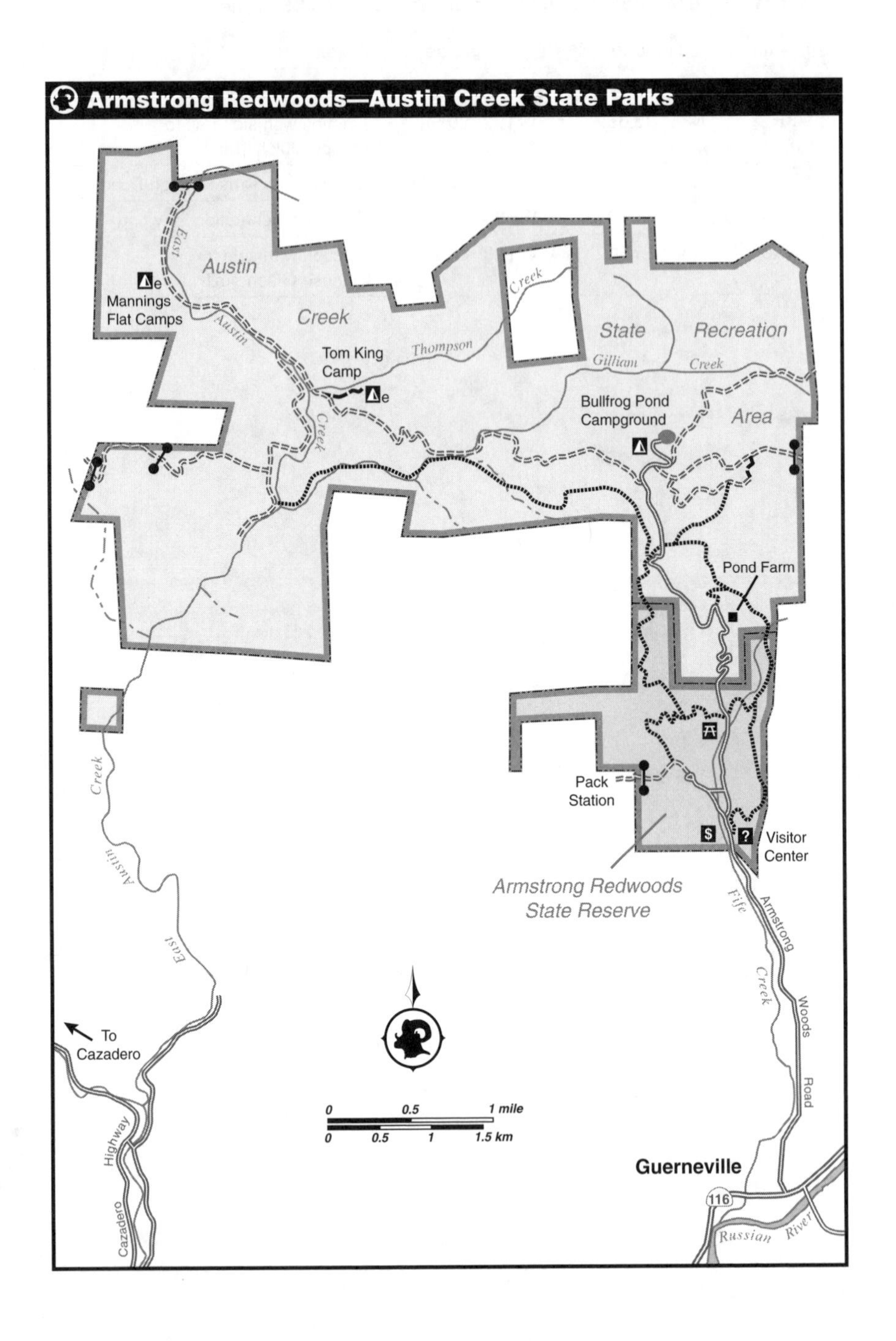
Armstrong Redwoods—Austin Creek State Parks
Austin Creek State Recreation Area
Mannings Flat Camps
Tom King Camp
East Austin Creek
Thompson
Creek
Gilliam Creek
Bullfrog Pond Campground
Pond Farm
Pack Station
Visitor Center
Armstrong Redwoods State Reserve
Fife Creek
Armstrong Woods Road
To Cazadero
Cazadero Highway
0 0.5 1 mile
0 0.5 1 1.5 km
Guerneville
116
Russian River

Chapter 5

Armstrong Redwoods State Natural Reserve

Armstrong Redwoods State Natural Reserve, 2 miles north of Guerneville, is home to Sonoma County's last major stand of old-growth redwoods. Here, you can gaze in wonder upon giants already ancient when Columbus discovered America—trees that were alive when Charlemagne conquered Europe nearly 1,300 years ago.

Until the last half of the 19th century, such redwood groves—many even more magnificent than Armstrong—were common throughout the Russian River area. Some trees stood nearly 400 feet tall and had been alive since before the dawn of Christianity. Today almost all of these majestic giants, the world's tallest living things, have fallen victim to the lumberjack's saw. Throughout the Pacific Northwest, less than 5 percent of the original old-growth forest still survives; in Sonoma County, besides Armstrong only a few small privately owned groves remain.

This 805-acre reserve gives you the rare opportunity to experience the stately grandeur of an ancient forest. To fully appreciate it, you'll have to get out of your car and walk. It isn't hard, for much of the park is level bottomland. Stand in awe of the towering redwoods, then study the complex understory illuminated by softly filtered sunlight. On the forest floor, notice the ground cover of pervasive, clover-like redwood sorrel. Then turn to the various ferns and wildflowers: trillium, calypso orchid, wild ginger, and fetid adder's tongue. Finally, observe the tanoaks, bay laurels, maples, and Douglas-firs that would, if not for the redwoods, dominate the landscape.

Armstrong is ideally suited for exploring the natural environment. Facilities include hiking trails, picnic areas, a large outdoor amphitheater, and a pack station where you can take guided horseback rides. This is also the entrance to Austin Creek State Recreation Area, a largely undeveloped region of hiking and riding trails with panoramic views of the surrounding wilderness. While there is no camping within Armstrong, a 23-site campground is situated above Bullfrog Pond in Austin Creek.

Getting There

From Santa Rosa, take Highway 101 to the River Road exit. Turn west and head 15 miles to the Russian River town of Guerneville. With the construction of a new highway bridge in 1997–98, Guerneville finally acquired not only its first, but also its second traffic light. The second

Redwood sorrel in bloom in Armstrong Redwoods.

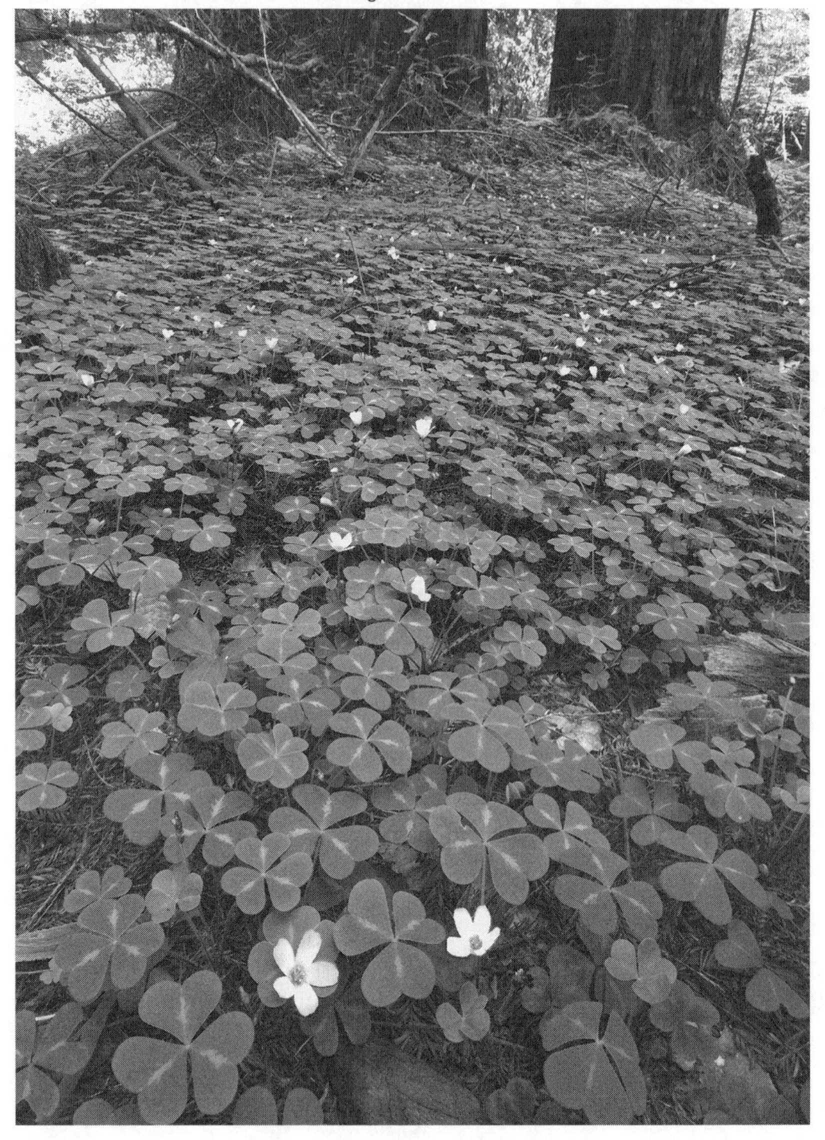

light is Armstrong Woods Road. Make a right turn here and drive 2.4 miles north to the park entrance. The visitor center and a parking lot are on your right just prior to the entrance station. You can park there (currently free), or you can pay the entrance fee and drive on into the park.

Natural Environment

The park lies along the drainage of Fife Creek as it descends toward the Russian River. This is a true old-growth redwood forest, with some trees as much as 1400 years old. The towering giants filter out much of the sunlight and keep down the competing vegetation. Lesser trees such as Douglas-firs, maples, and bay trees flourish only at the edges of the forest. Shade-tolerant tanoaks are one of the few species that can thrive under the redwood canopy.

Some of the forest near the park entrance was logged in the late 1800s, so the trees there are second-growth redwoods. Many have sprouted from the roots of the old stumps, forming "fairy rings" of smaller trees around the stumps. These are not new trees, but rather new growths from the old tree. Redwoods are one of the few conifers that can sprout from existing tree roots as well as from seed. In an old-growth forest such as this, most regeneration occurs from sprouts rather than seeds.

Armstrong's popularity has become a threat to its continued health. Throngs of visitors trample the countryside daily, compacting the soil and destroying the natural ground cover. Redwoods are especially susceptible to this abuse, for despite their enormous height, they do not have a taproot to lend stability. Instead, their shallow root system spreads out just under the surface for as much as 100 feet in all directions. If the root system is damaged, the tree can topple in a strong wind. Redwoods also depend on the forest's thick natural humus layer to retain vital moisture. The effects of a century of heavy use are slowly taking their toll.

The grove's fragile nature was recognized as early as the 1960s. In 1964 its status was changed from State Park to State Reserve. Camping was no longer permitted and visitors were encouraged to remain on established trails. In recent years a series of wooden fences has been erected along the trails to further discourage cross-country travel. As you explore this delicate grove, please stay on established trails and try not to disturb the forest floor.

History

California's gold rush in the mid-1800s led to a period of enormous growth in the San Francisco Bay Area. Throughout the region, lumber was urgently needed for new construction, and the vast tracts of redwoods north of the Bay were a primary resource. The Russian River area was at the forefront of this "lumber rush."

In 1860, R. B. Lunsford began a logging operation along the river at a site called "Big Bottom." The surrounding forest was soon mowed down and the village that grew among the stumps became informally known as "Stumptown." Others soon followed Lunsford, and sawmills sprang up all along the river. By 1870, the largest mill was owned by Thomas Heald and George Guerne. Stumptown's residents decided their town needed a more respectable name, and since the town of Healdsburg was already named for Thomas' brother Harmon, they settled on the new name of "Guerneville" (the middle "e" is silent).

Three miles north of town lay a dense, forested valley. The local Indians called it "The Dark Place" and considered it haunted. Thomas Stone and A. E. Laud, undaunted by the Indians' tales, staked out claims in the densest part of the forest at the site of today's park. The two evidently held the land only as an investment, for they did not cut any timber and soon sold it. The land changed hands several more times before finally being purchased by Col. James B. Armstrong in 1874.

Colonel Armstrong had been born in Ohio on August 20, 1824. Trained as a surveyor, he also served as a newspaper reporter, county treasurer, and delegate to the 1860 Republican National Convention before joining the Union Army during the Civil War. In his first term of duty, he was captured during the Battle of Richmond, Kentucky, but soon made a daring escape. (Details of his escape are described in his definitive biography, *Colonel James B. Armstrong, His Family and His Legacy*, by Carmen J. Finley and Doris M. Dickenson, published in 2008 by Stewards of the Coast and Redwoods.) In 1864 he re-enlisted as a full colonel, but saw no action during his 100-day term of enlistment.

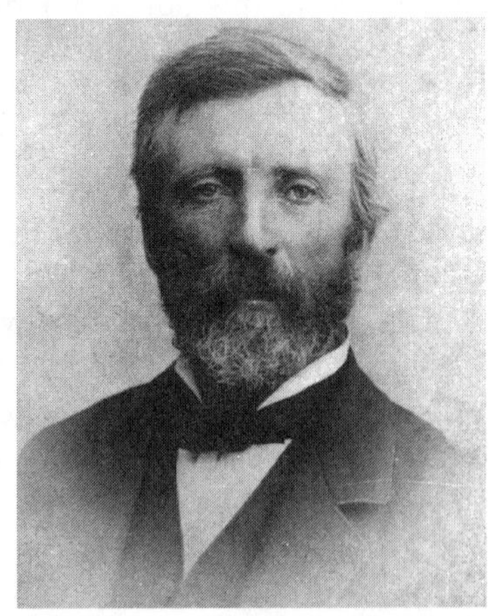

Colonel James B. Armstrong, 1824–1900. Photo taken in 1883. (Photo courtesy of Armstrong Redwoods State Reserve.)

Colonel Armstrong moved his family to California in 1874. Both his wife, Eleanor, and daughter, Kate, were in poor health, and he hoped the California climate would help. (The move didn't help much. Eleanor died in 1880 and Kate in 1898.)

A shrewd businessman, Armstrong purchased timberlands throughout the Guerneville area and set up a lumber mill capable of producing 30,000 board feet per day. He prospered not only in lumber, but also in real estate. As his lands were cleared of trees, he subdivided and sold them. As a close friend of the horticulturist Luther Burbank, he particularly encouraged buyers to plant fruit trees on their lands.

Many people viewed the redwoods as an inexhaustible supply of timber, but Armstrong recognized they wouldn't last forever. In 1891 he proposed that his Guerneville grove be purchased by the State and set aside as a public park. He even donated $100,000 to help the cause. But some skeptics claimed the trees had rotten hearts and he stood to gain more by selling it as a park than by logging it. The proposal bogged down in the legislature. Worn down by a series of financial misfortunes, Armstrong gave up. He died in 1900.

The fight to save the grove was then picked up by his daughter Lizzie and her husband, the Reverend William Ladd Jones, popularly known as "Parson Jones." The two worked with State Assemblyman Harrison M. LeBaron and State Senator Walter Price. The legislature passed a bill to purchase the grove in 1909, but Governor James Gillette was unconvinced. It was an election year, and Gillette vetoed what he considered just another spending measure. Parson Jones died the following year. As a memorial, Lizzie named a tree in the park for him and another for her father.

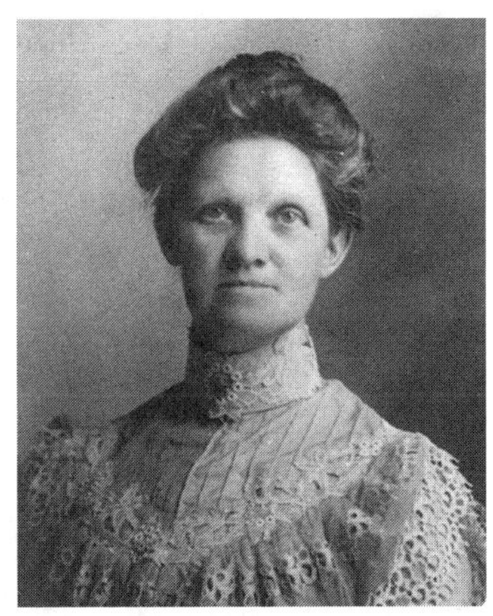

Lizzie Armstrong Jones, 1850–1924. (Photo courtesy of Armstrong Redwoods State Reserve.)

Lizzie would not give up. Working with Senator Price, she tried again in 1916. This time the plan was to make it a county park rather than trying to convince the entire State. With the help of a committee of dignitaries and hundreds of volunteers, she put together a well-organized campaign. Decorated cars with blaring horns paraded throughout the county. Newspaper editorials were

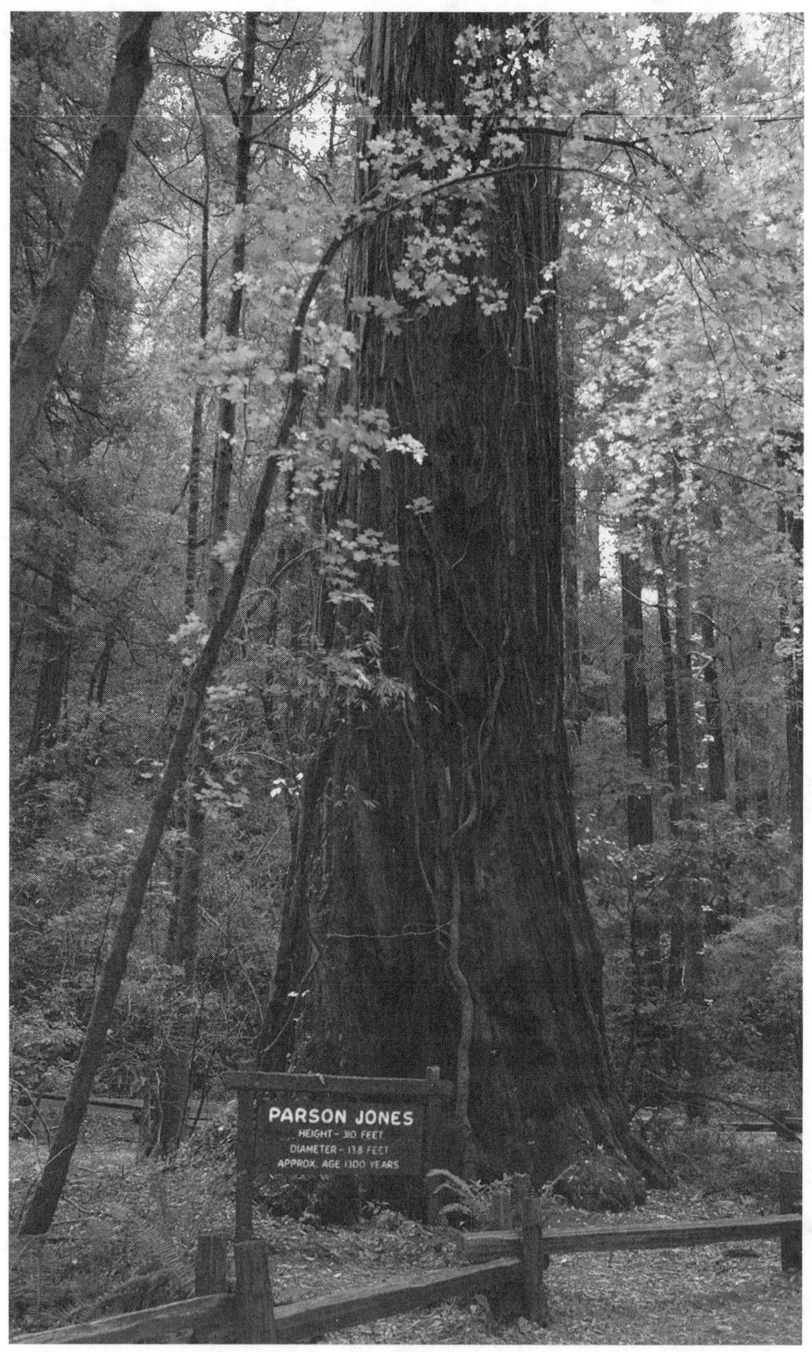
PARSON JONES
HEIGHT - 310 FEET
DIAMETER - 13.8 FEET
APPROX. AGE 1300 YEARS

The Parson Jones Tree is over 1,300 years old and is the tallest tree in the park.

unanimous in support, and when the votes were counted the measure passed by nearly a two-to-one margin. The park remained county property until 1934, when it was acquired by the State as part of the purchase of Sonoma Coast State Beach.

Facilities

Visitor Center and Parking Area

You'll see the visitor center adjacent to a large parking area on your right, just before the park's entrance kiosk. It's open 10 A.M.–4 P.M. on weekends and holidays, staffed by state park volunteers. Here, you can see posters and exhibits that portray the park's history and natural environment. You can also buy a number of relevant books and postcards.

At the parking lot you'll also find restrooms and the ranger station. Both this lot and the visitor center lie outside the reserve's current fee area, but if you do park here, consider stopping at the visitor center and contributing something to the donation box. It's a small price to pay to help keep this magnificent treasure open for future generations to enjoy. If you do decide to drive on into the park, you will need to stop at the kiosk and pay the entrance fee.

Redwood Forest Theater

The historic Redwood Forest Theater lies nestled in a hollow surrounded by towering redwoods. It has an elevated stage and rows

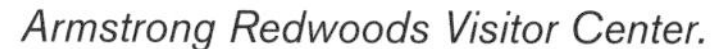
Armstrong Redwoods Visitor Center.

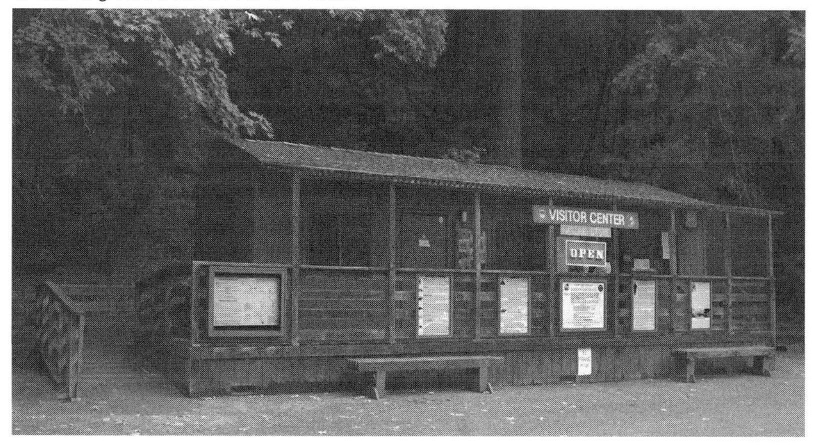

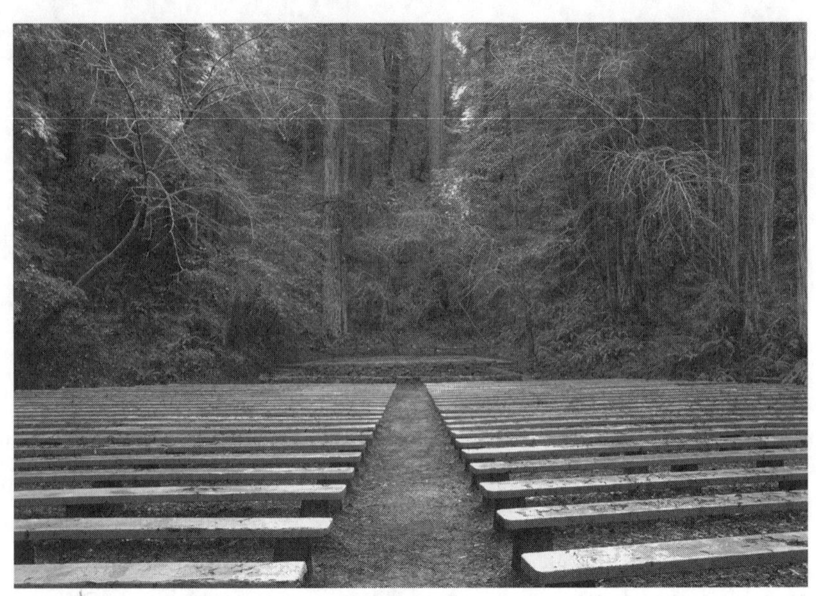

Redwood Forest Theater.

of wooden bench seats capable of seating over a thousand people. In earlier days it was used for such events as theatrical performances and weddings. The author and his wife were fortunate enough to be married here in 1976, but it was closed to weddings a few years later. In recent years, the Parks Department has sponsored a series of public performances in the theater during the summer months as a benefit for the local cooperating association, the Stewards of the Coast and Redwoods. Check the Stewards' website at www.stewardsofthecoastandredwoods.org for current information.

WPA-affiliated work crews built the theater during the Great Depression. Construction began in 1934 and the theater was dedicated on Sunday, September 27, 1936. A reported crowd of 3,000 people celebrated the dedication that day.

Today, you're likely to have the theater nearly to yourself, especially if you visit on a weekday. On occasion, you may be joined by a family with energetic children or perhaps a solitary figure meditating in silence.

To reach the theater, park in the lot adjacent to the Colonel Armstrong Tree. Walk part way around the loop road to the marked trail heading west. Continue a level 0.1-mile to the theater. There are no picnic tables here, but you can easily spread out among the benches. There is a dual restroom with running water along the path to the theater.

Pack Station

A privately run pack station is 0.5 mile beyond the Armstrong Tree parking area, on private property at the edge of the park. Take the one-lane dirt road (closed 5 P.M.–10 A.M.) and follow the signposts to the camp. This private concession, licensed by the State, offers guided horseback rides for all levels of experience. Advance reservations are required. You can choose from a variety of rides ranging from a two-hour tour to a multi-day pack trip. Guide-owners Jonathan and Laura Ayers conduct the tours, complete with gourmet meals and nature talks. Call 707-887-2939 for more information, or check their web page at http://redwoodhorses.com.

Picnic Area

The large picnic area is 0.8 mile up Armstrong Woods Road from the entrance station. Picnic sites lie along a loop road branching left from the main road just before it climbs up the canyon into Austin Creek. You'll find tables, barbeque facilities, and restrooms here. At the head of the loop road, adjacent to the restrooms, lies the trailhead for Pool Ridge Spur Trail. This steep path connects with Pool Ridge Trail after climbing 400 feet in less than a half mile.

An adjacent group picnic area with separate parking can be reserved through the park office. Another large parking lot and picnic area sit just north of the group picnic area. The steep spur trail to East Ridge Trail departs from the end of this lot.

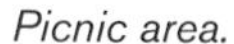

Picnic area.

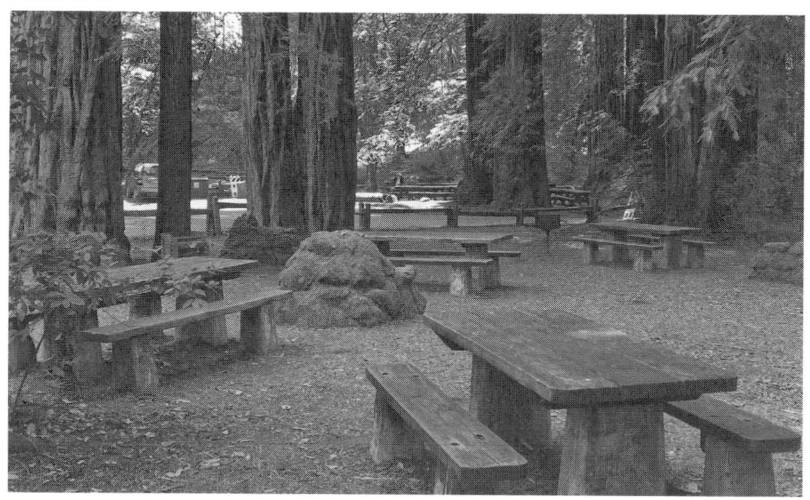

Armstrong Woods Trails

Several trails run through the park, passing numerous points of interest along the way. Pioneer Trail—Discovery Trail Loop is an easy walk. Discovery Trail has been specially designed to meet the needs of visually impaired visitors, but can be enjoyed by everyone. Portions of the Pioneer Trail have been developed as a self-guided nature trail, with markers and descriptive signs at various points along the way to explain the basics of forest ecology. Be sure to pick up a copy of the descriptive nature trail guide at the visitor center.

Pool Ridge Trail and East Ridge Trail are more physically challenging. They climb hundreds of feet as they emerge from the forest shadows and continue up the exposed ridges of Austin Creek. These two trails are described in the next chapter on Austin Creek.

Trail 22: Pioneer Trail-Discovery Trail Loop

Length: 1.6 miles round trip, 1 hour

Difficulty: Easy–portions are disabled accessible

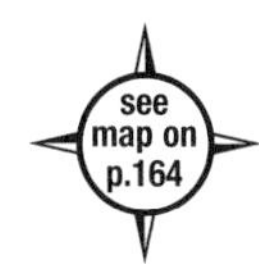

Overview: This level loop trail takes you through the heart of an old-growth redwood forest, with a side trip to the Forest Theater. You climb only 50 feet the entire way, making this an easy hike through redwood forest. Interpretive signs along the way explain such topics as forest animals, Native Americans, and methods of redwood regeneration. The disabled-accessible Discovery Trail to the Colonel Armstrong Tree has several features designed to aid visually impaired persons.

Directions to Trailhead: From the town of Guerneville, take Armstrong Woods Road 2.4 miles north to the Armstrong Woods entrance station. The visitor center parking area is on your right just prior to the entrance station. Currently, this parking area is free of charge. If there is space, park here. Otherwise, park along Armstrong Woods Road. Walk to the ranger kiosk on the north side of the parking area. The Pioneer Trail trailhead is left of the road just past the kiosk.

Trail Description. From the trailhead to the left of the ranger kiosk, follow the trail through the redwood forest. Sword ferns, bracken ferns, redwood sorrel, tanoaks, and a small amount of poison oak cover the forest floor. In 500 feet, look for a group of four redwoods clustered together on your left. A fallen tree here provides your first opportunity to study the redwood's complex root structure.

The trail crosses the road near the Parson Jones Tree at 0.1 mile. Towering 310 feet above the forest floor, Parson Jones is the tallest redwood in the park. It was given its name by Colonel Armstrong's daughter, Lizzie, after she married the Reverend William Ladd Jones in 1901. It is estimated to be over 1,300 years old. Note the thick vines of poison oak clinging tightly up its trunk.

Just past the Parson Jones Tree, you come to a display of the cross-section of a redwood that germinated in the year A.D. 948. Labels on the tree show the dates of various historical events in relation to the tree's rings. About 100 feet farther on, a large fairy ring on the right is known as Cathedral Ring. The trees forming this circle have all sprouted from the roots of a single central tree that fell many generations ago. From the size of this ring it is possible that the current trees represent more than one generation of successive sproutings.

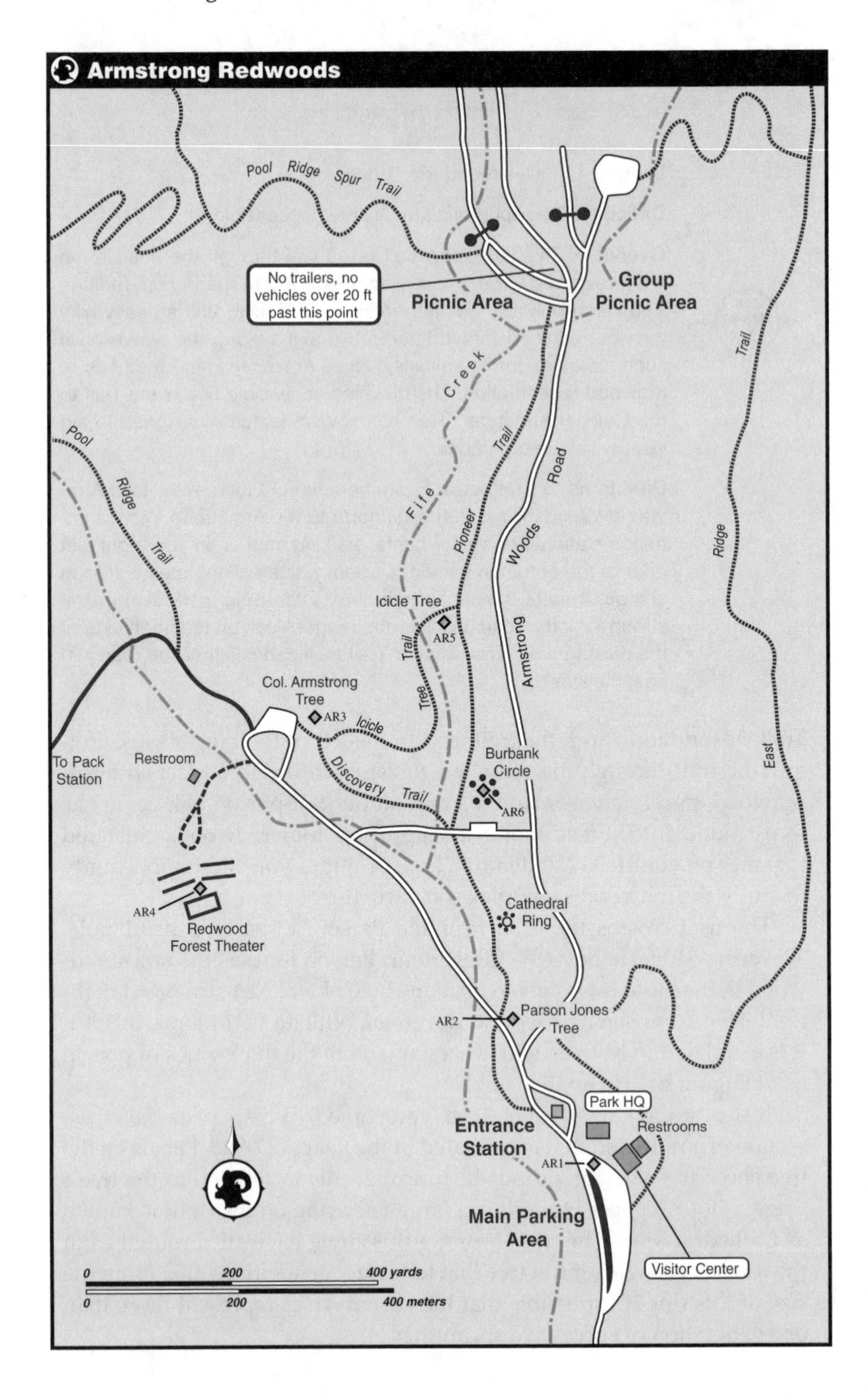
Armstrong Redwoods
Pool Ridge Spur Trail
No trailers, no vehicles over 20 ft past this point
Picnic Area
Group Picnic Area
Fife Creek Trail
Pioneer Trail
Armstrong Woods Road
East Ridge Trail
Pool Ridge Trail
Icicle Tree
AR5
Icicle Tree Trail
Col. Armstrong Tree
AR3
Discovery Trail
To Pack Station
Restroom
Burbank Circle
AR6
AR4
Redwood Forest Theater
Cathedral Ring
AR2
Parson Jones Tree
Park HQ
Entrance Station
Restrooms
AR1
Main Parking Area
Visitor Center
0
200
400 yards
0
200
400 meters

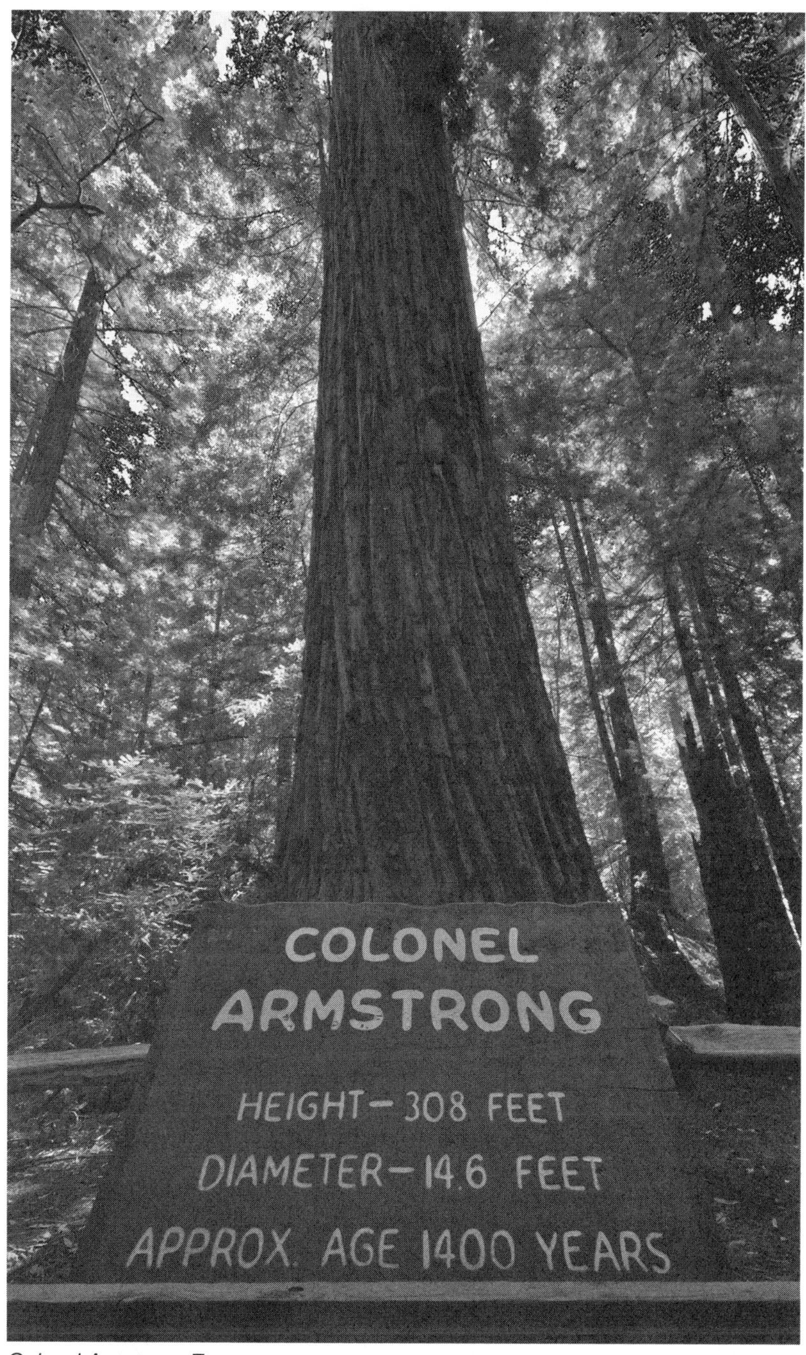

Colonel Armstrong Tree.

You pass another fallen tree with a gnarled root on your left at 0.2 mile and reach a connecting road at 0.3 mile. Pioneer Trail, which will serve as your return path, continues straight ahead, but for this hike, turn left and take the road a short distance to where Discovery Trail branches off to the right. This disabled-accessible trail includes a wire cable running the length of a wooden railing to help guide visually-impaired visitors along the trail. Numerous bronze plaques in English and Braille describe trailside features. At one spot along the way, a wooden ramp has been built right up to the side of a tree so that visitors can feel and smell the redwood bark without damaging its delicate roots.

You reach the Colonel Armstrong Tree at 0.5 mile. This is the most massive tree in the Reserve and was named by Lizzie Armstrong Jones after her late father. Although its 308-foot height is 2 feet shorter than the Parson Jones Tree, its 14.6-foot diameter is nearly a foot larger. It could be as much as 100 years older than Parson Jones.

After admiring the Colonel Armstrong Tree, head over to the adjacent parking area, then back down the road a short distance to the Forest Theater trailhead on your right at 0.6 mile. As you follow this trail, look for a bronze plaque on your left, mounted to a rock slab adjacent to an enormous redwood. It honors Robert S. Coon, the park's first caretaker, appointed by the county on July 1, 1917.

You pass a dual restroom with flush toilets and running water on your right. Just beyond is a Y junction. Take the right fork to reach Forest Theater at 0.7 mile. You may want to take a short break here to admire the stately surroundings or enjoy a picnic lunch. Then walk down the center aisle between the rows of wooden benches, capable of seating over a thousand people. The wood for these benches was gathered outside the park at Guernewood Park. The current benches were installed in 1951.

Just before reaching the stage, turn left and exit the theater on a side path that connects back with the main trail near the restrooms. Return the way you came to the Colonel Armstrong Tree. Just before you get there, look to the right of the trail at the parking lot to see an unpretentious bronze plaque mounted on a granite slab. It is dedicated to the memory of Lizzie Armstrong Jones, the woman whose untiring efforts almost singlehandedly brought the park into being. She died in 1924 at age 74.

After passing the Colonel Armstrong Tree, take the trail that heads left toward the picnic area. This is Icicle Tree Trail. It traverses the northwest side of a ravine along Fife Creek. At 1.0 mile, you descend a series of wooden steps and pass beside a redwood with a hollow center known as a "goosepen," formed when the center of the tree was burned out by fire. Pioneers built fences around hollows like these to keep poultry and other small farm animals. Continuing on, look for a large fallen redwood on your left with great strips of bark lying on the ground beneath it.

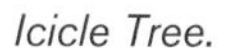
Icicle Tree.

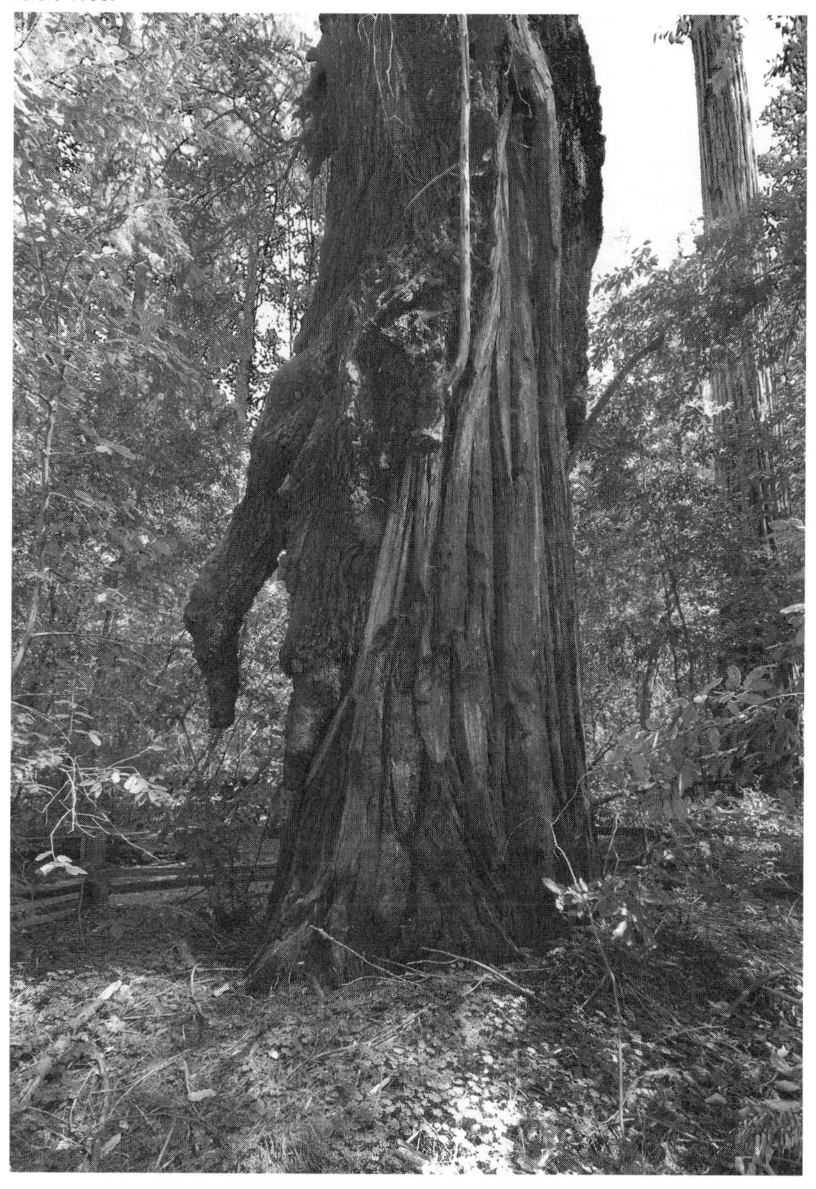

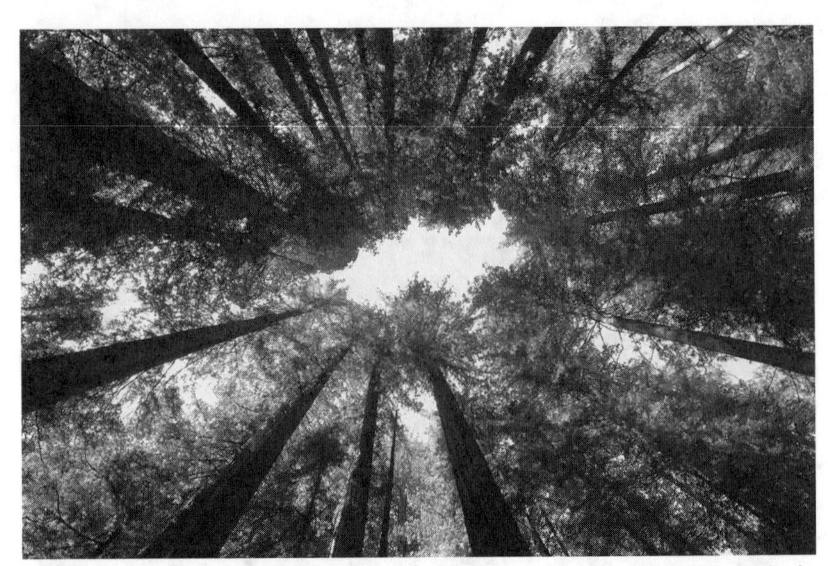

No one knows whether Burbank Circle is an enormous fairy ring or just the result of a natural distribution of sproutings.

The trail curves right and crosses a wooden bridge over Fife Creek just before reaching Icicle Tree at 1.1 mile. The large nodules growing on the side of this tree's trunk are redwood burls. These dormant masses of buds can grow into fantastic shapes, stirring the imagination to conjure up visions of strange faces or animals. Although they appear similar to cancer in humans, burls are not harmful to the tree. Burls are prized by collectors, who craft them into beautiful tables. Most of the long, icicle-shaped burls that once grew from this tree were cut and carried away by vandals, leaving only the less exotic shapes you see now behind.

Continuing past Icicle Tree, you quickly reach the junction with Pioneer Trail. The picnic area lies to the left, an optional 0.6-mile round-trip hike. If you choose not to hike to the picnic area, turn left and follow Pioneer Trail back toward the park entrance. You soon pass a Douglas-fir on your left and more redwoods with large burls protruding from their sides. Two redwoods with goosepens stand side-by-side nearby.

You reach Burbank Circle at 1.2 miles. This circle of redwoods appears to be an enormous fairy ring far larger than any other known example. Not everyone agrees that it is, in fact, a true fairy ring, for no roots from a single large tree can be found. It could be the result of a natural distribution of seed cones, or perhaps even the work of ancient shamans in the tradition of Stonehenge or Easter Island.

After leaving Burbank Circle you return to the junction at the connecting road. Cross the road and retrace your steps along Pioneer Trail to the Parson Jones tree at 1.4 miles and the visitor center at 1.6 miles.

Trail 22: Pioneer Trail–Discovery Loop Trail Waypoints (WGS84 Datum)

Name	Latitude	Longitude	Feature
AR1	N38° 31.940′	W123° 00.162′	Visitor Center parking lot
AR2	N38° 32.045′	W123° 00.245′	Parson Jones Tree
AR3	N38° 32.225′	W123° 00.427′	Colonel Armstrong Tree
AR4	N38° 32.156′	W123° 00.559′	Redwood Forest Theater
AR5	N38° 32.310′	W123° 00.284′	Icicle Tree
AR6	N38° 32.176′	W123° 00.272′	Burbank Circle

Armstrong Redwoods—Austin Creek State Parks

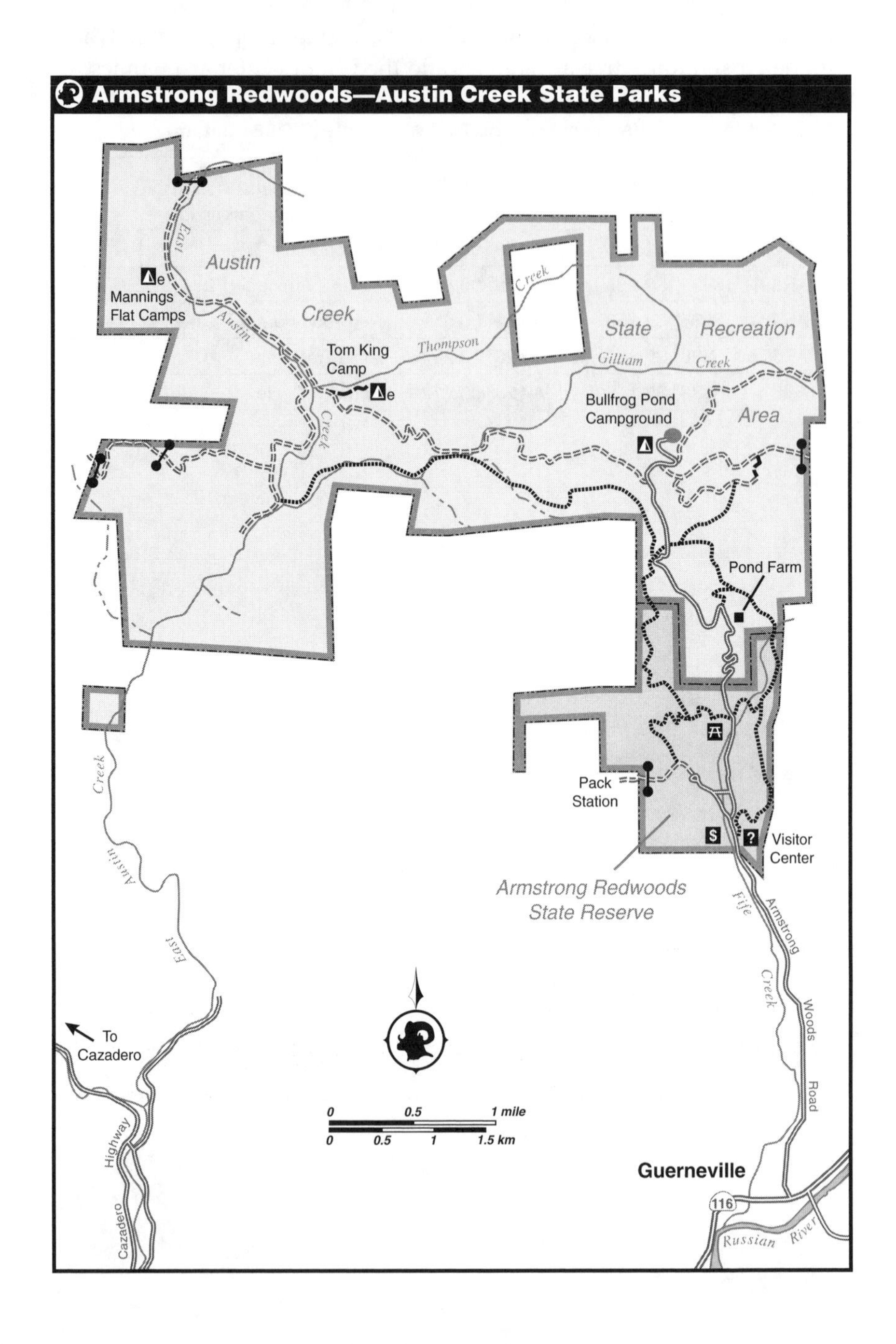

Chapter 6

Austin Creek State Recreation Area

The grassy, oak-covered hillsides of Austin Creek State Recreation Area are a far cry from the sheltered redwood forest in nearby Armstrong Redwoods. Austin Creek's 5,600 acres offer spectacular wilderness views along 20 miles of undulating trails. Much of the area is accessible only on foot or horseback, and as a result, it is one of the least-visited parks in the region.

Getting There

To get to Austin Creek you must drive through Armstrong Redwoods State Reserve. Take Armstrong Woods Road from Guerneville to the entrance station, pay the fee, and bear right a few hundred feet later. Drive 0.7 mile to the picnic area, then take the narrow, one-lane road that climbs uphill toward the left. Vehicles longer than 20 feet and vehicles with trailers are not permitted on this road. (If you have a motor home or horse trailer, you should park in the main lot at the entrance to Armstrong Redwoods.)

As you climb the canyon you leave the redwood reserve and enter Austin Creek State Recreation Area. This two-way road has several

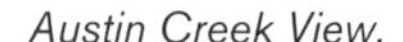
Austin Creek View.

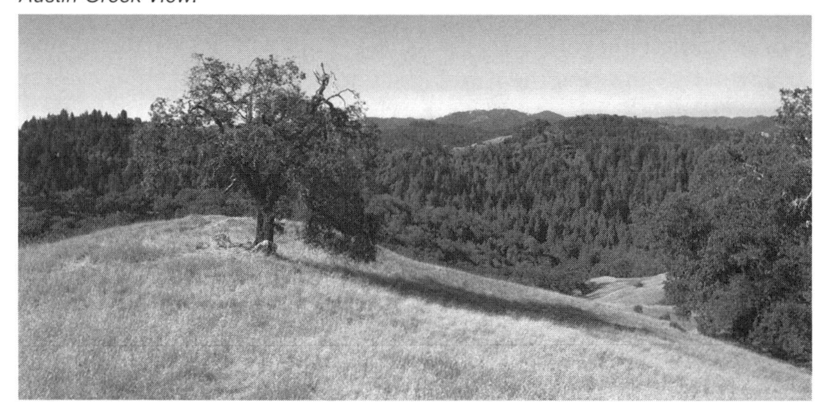

switchbacks with limited visibility, especially for uphill drivers. Take it slow and watch for downhill traffic. If you meet a car coming down at a spot where you can't pass, the downhill car must back up to a safe spot and let the uphill traffic pass.

Natural Environment

The park is a sprawling mass of hills and valleys with few level spots. Live oaks, tanoaks, interior oaks, firs, and madrones cover most of the sloping terrain. Manzanita and scrub oaks grow in the driest regions, while bay laurels, maples, and alders grow in the canyons. In spring and summer, extensive wildflower displays of California poppies, lupines, Indian paintbrushes, shooting stars, and Douglas irises blanket the hillsides.

Some of the animals found in the park include deer, raccoons, skunks, squirrels, and an occasional fox, coyote, or bobcat. In recent years mountain lions have made a comeback, though they are still rare. Black bear have also been sighted on occasion. Feral pigs descended from domestic animals are fairly common in the park.

Birds you'll see in the park include California quail, ravens, black-shouldered kites, wood ducks, spotted owls, and the ubiquitous turkey vulture soaring high overhead. Hawks, great blue herons, and woodpeckers are also common, and on occasion you may encounter a flock of wild turkeys as you hike the trails.

Sunfish and black bass can be found in Bullfrog Pond, while trout and salmon live in the streams. With a valid California fishing license you can fish at Bullfrog Pond, but all streams are closed to protect vital spawning habitats.

Rattlesnakes can sometimes be seen along the park's trails, so stay alert, especially in warm weather. If you are fortunate enough to encounter a snake, keep your distance and don't make any sudden moves. Rattlesnakes are normally reclusive, but will strike if threatened. You won't always hear the warning sound of rattles first, but if you do, the reverberating echoes will be an experience you won't soon forget.

This is also tick country, so use a suitable repellent and check yourself after every hike. Lyme disease, although not common, is found in ticks throughout Northern California.

Austin Creek's climate is hotter and drier than Armstrong Redwoods. While Armstrong is blanketed in summer fog, Austin Creek's ridges often remain exposed to the sun. Summer temperatures commonly exceed 100°F, while winter nights sometimes drop below freezing. Winter storms have been known to leave a dusting of snow on the hills.

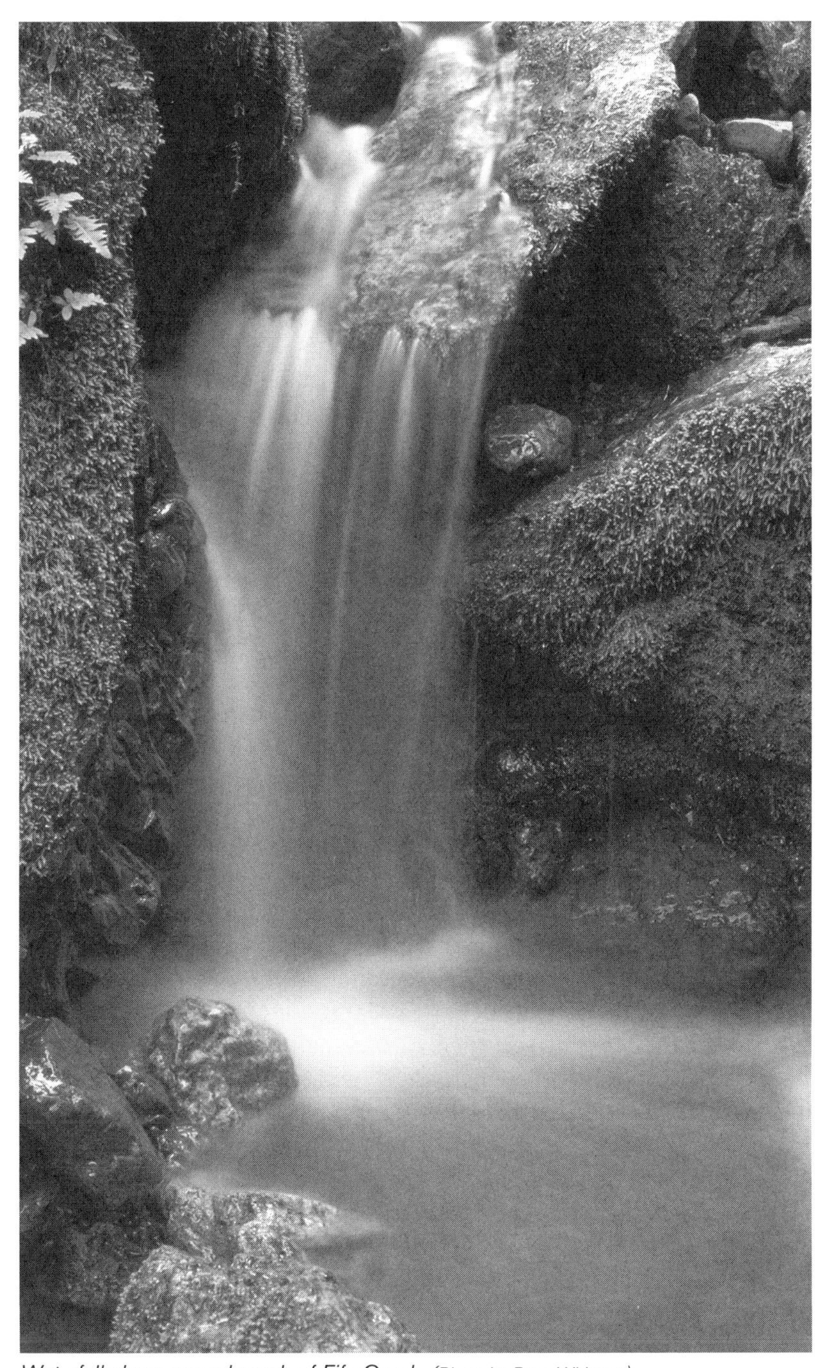

Waterfall along upper branch of Fife Creek. (Photo by Russ Whitman)

History

No Native American villages are known to have existed within the present park boundaries, though the land was almost certainly used for hunting, fishing, and acorn gathering. Early white settlers also tended to avoid the rolling hillsides in favor of more easily cultivated lands in the valleys below. There are, however, remnants of several early homesteads in the form of old orchards, gardens, and a few houses or foundations scattered around the park. Some of the newer houses now serve as residences for park staff.

The first major development occurred in the late 1800s when a magnesite mine was established northwest of the park at Red Slide. To get the ore to Guerneville a county road was built for mule teams and wagons. Originally known as Magnesite Road and Panorama Grade, parts of this road now form East Austin Creek Trail. Vehicular traffic is no longer permitted, though mountain bikes are allowed.

The mule teams were eventually replaced by a 2-foot narrow-gauge railroad that followed the west side of East Austin Creek. The mine closed in the 1920s and the tracks were removed about 10 years later. Though time has reclaimed much of the old railroad grade, you can still see traces of it in spots, including an occasional timber from an old trestle.

A one-room schoolhouse, Summit School, once stood on Gilliam Ridge at a parking area about halfway between the trailheads for Gilliam Creek Trail and East Austin Creek Trail. The exact site of the school is no longer known. Even a group of alumni who gathered for a reunion some years ago couldn't agree on the location.

In 1939, architect Gordon Herr and his wife, the writer Jane Herr, bought 160 acres of the Walker Ranch just north of Armstrong Redwoods. Longtime patrons of the arts, they christened their ranch "Pond Farm" and founded what became a world-renowned artistic community. Bauhaus-trained potter Marguerite Wildenhain came in 1942 to escape Nazi persecution. Her husband Franz, conscripted by the Wehrmacht, joined her in 1947. Others who came over the years included sculptor Claire Falkenstein, weaver Trude Guermonprez, metalworkers Viktor Ries and Harry Dixon, and frescoists Lucienne Bloch and Stephen Pope Dimitroff.

Students flocked from around the world to learn from the masters. Summers were spent teaching these aspiring artists. As described in the school's course catalog, "Pond Farm is a place where craftsmen live. Working individually but with the same basic concept as to professional and artistic standards, they have formed a group—the Pond Farm Workshops. The school offers students the opportunity to

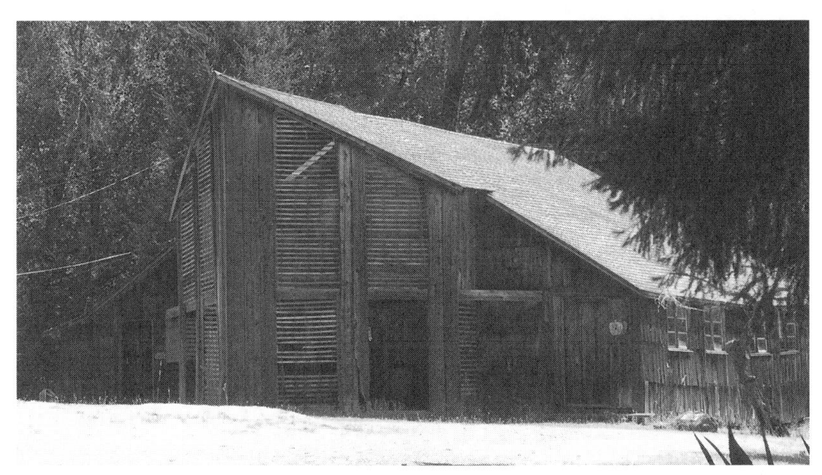

For many years this barn at Pond Farm was the studio for acclaimed potter Marguerite Wildenhain. It is now closed to the public.

serve an apprenticeship under the artists of this group." Many courses were taught at the Hexagon House near the entrance to Armstrong Redwoods. (The unique building, designed and built by Gordon Herr in 1948, was destroyed by fire in 1991.) Years later, local historian and newspaper columnist Gaye LeBaron cited Pond Farm as "the beginning of art in the Bay Area."

The Herrs found it difficult to keep the strong personalities of the artists in check. Constant bickering wore everyone down, and when Jane died of cancer in 1952, Gordon lost interest in the project. The group quickly dispersed, with only potter Marguerite Wildenhain remaining. She lived at Pond Farm until her death in 1985. She continued to teach and throw pots at the farm well into her 80s. Her house and barn, closed to the public, remain along Armstrong Woods Road.

Much of what is now parkland was purchased by developers who envisioned damming East Austin Creek and creating an exclusive subdivision. When this proved infeasible the land was sold to Santa Rosa-based Lumbermen's Leasing Corporation, whose development plans were also thwarted. The corporation then proposed selling the land to the State as a wilderness park. The deal included a plan to acquire adjoining parcels by eminent domain from landowners who were not informed until after the legislation was passed. The 4,000 acres owned by Lumbermen's Leasing Corp. was purchased in 1964, but the remaining parcels took several more years and a series of court actions to acquire. As part of the agreement to purchase Marguerite Wildenhain's property, she was allowed to live on the site for the remainder of her life.

Facilities

Bullfrog Pond Campground

Older maps show the reservoir here as "Redwood Lake." The name was changed long ago after one too many expectant camper arrived with boat in tow, expecting the "lake" to be big enough for aquatic recreation. It is the product of an earthen dam built by an early settler. The campground consists of 23 sites in a wooded setting on the hill above the pond. A camp host is on duty much of the year. Sites are available year-round on a first-come, first-serve basis. Register at the Armstrong Redwoods entrance station.

Each site has a table, food locker, and fire ring. Flush toilets and potable water are also provided, but there are no showers. Keep your food either in the lockers or in your vehicle to prevent raccoons from enjoying a nocturnal feast.

You may fish in Bullfrog Pond if you have a valid California fishing license. Remember that fishing is not permitted in streams within the park. The secluded setting, far from city lights, also makes this an ideal spot for stargazing on clear nights.

Backcountry Camps

Hikers and horseback riders may wish to camp at either of two backcountry camps. Campers must obtain a backcountry permit and pay a fee at the Armstrong Redwoods entrance station. Be warned that the camps lie 3–4 miles from their trailheads along hikes that descend 1,000 to 1,300 feet. The return trip is much more exhausting than the outbound hike.

Even if you don't plan to stay overnight, carry plenty of water and snacks, and think twice about venturing out during the heat of summer.

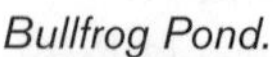

Bullfrog Pond.

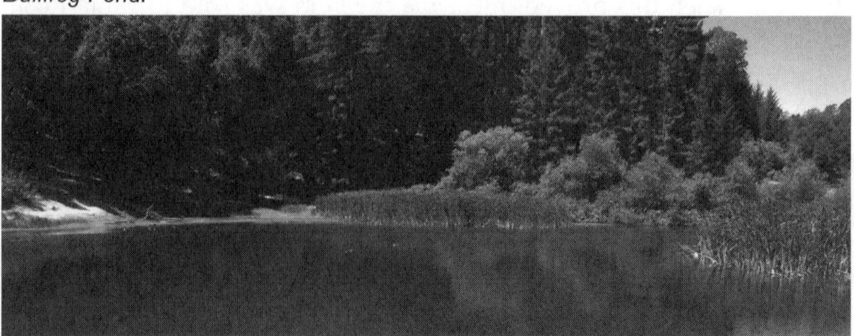

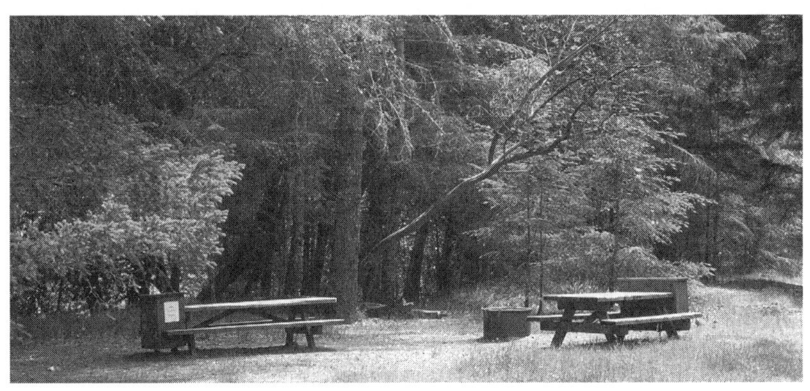

Mannings Flat Trail Camp. (Photo by Russ Whitman)

Always check at the ranger station to learn about any trail closures or fire danger before starting out. Ground fires are prohibited during periods of extreme fire danger. You should also keep a watchful eye out for rattlesnakes along the trail at any time of year.

Tom King Camp. At 3.1 miles from the trailhead, this is the closer of the two backcountry camps. It lies in a shaded area along Thompson Creek, down a short spur trail from East Austin Creek Trail. Facilities include two picnic tables, fire rings, and an outhouse. If you don't bring your own water you must treat the creek water by microfiltration, by boiling, or with iodine tablets.

Begin your hike by parking at the overlook parking lot just past the East Austin Creek trailhead. Hike down the trail 2.8 miles to the spur trail on your right. The camp lies 0.3 mile up the spur trail.

Mannings Flat Camp. This site lies along the old magnesite railroad, 4.1 miles from the East Austin Creek Trailhead. You can still see sections of the railroad grade and remnants of a trestle south of the camp. Two campsites lie along the creek in the shade of trees adjacent to a large meadow. Another two sites lie in a grove of oak and fir trees 0.1 mile farther down the trail. Each area has two picnic tables with food lockers, fire rings, a trash can, horse hitching rails, and an outhouse. Bring your own water or be prepared to treat the creek water before drinking. Use the lockers to protect your food from raccoons or the occasional wild pig foraging through the camp.

Follow the directions for Tom King Camp, but instead of turning right at the junction, continue along East Austin Creek Trail. The last mile of the hike after crossing Thompson Creek Bridge is fairly level. You must ford East Austin Creek just before reaching the camp.

Austin Creek State Recreation Area Hiking Trails

Austin Creek is a hiker's and equestrian's paradise. Two dozen miles of trails give you views of forested glades and grand vistas. Spring is especially inviting, with brimming creeks and lush green hills covered with wildflowers. Temperatures are still mild, unlike the 100^{+}-degree temperatures at the height of summer.

Regardless of what time of year you venture out, carry plenty of water or be prepared to purify the water you find in streams. Remember that Gilliam Creek Trail and East Austin Creek Trail both descend sharply for the first couple of miles, so allow three times as long for your return trip as for your hike out.

Mountain bikes are permitted on paved roads and on service roads as shown on the map. They are not permitted on single-track trails. Check with rangers for current regulations before you ride.

Trail 23: East Austin Creek–Gilliam Creek Loop Trail

Length: 12 miles round trip, 6–8 hours; a shorter, 3.8-mile loop is possible by crossing from East Austin Creek Trail to Gilliam Creek Trail at the junction with Gilliam Creek, but this does not avoid most of the elevation change.

Difficulty: Strenuous

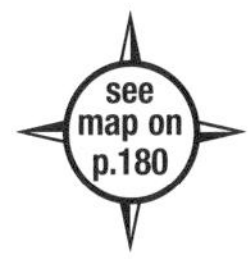

Overview: This challenging hike takes you through some of the most beautiful backcountry in the region. You descend 1000 feet during the first 1.5 miles of the hike and climb the same amount near the end, so be in good shape and bring plenty of food and water. Before attempting this hike, first check with the rangers at the Armstrong Woods entrance kiosk. This trail includes numerous fords of Gilliam Creek and East Austin Creek, and in wet weather, they may be impassible. In the dry season, all open flame may be prohibited, and in the worst conditions, the trail may be completely closed. Two hike-in backcountry camps are available for overnight stays; you must first obtain a permit at the Armstrong Woods entrance kiosk. Mountain bikes are permitted on the broad fire road of East Austin Creek Trail, but not on any of the single-track trails in the park.

Directions to Trailhead: From the town of Guerneville, take Armstrong Woods Road 2.4 miles north to the Armstrong Woods entrance station. Pay the entrance fee and enter the park. At the first road junction, take the right fork toward the picnic area. Drive 0.6 mile to the picnic area and then continue along the narrow, single-lane road that climbs uphill to your left. Continue another 2.2 miles to a large gravel parking area on your left, just before the Bullfrog Pond Campground. Drive cautiously along this road, as there are many blind curves with no room to pass oncoming cars except at occasional turnouts. According to law, when two cars meet and are unable to pass, the car traveling downhill must back up to the nearest safe spot and allow the uphill traffic to pass.

Trail Description. The trail departs between two concrete picnic tables at the west end of the parking area. Although unmarked here, this is Vista Point Trail. Follow the single-track path down the grass-covered side of the ridge. East Austin Creek Trail, your eventual destination, is visible below on your left.

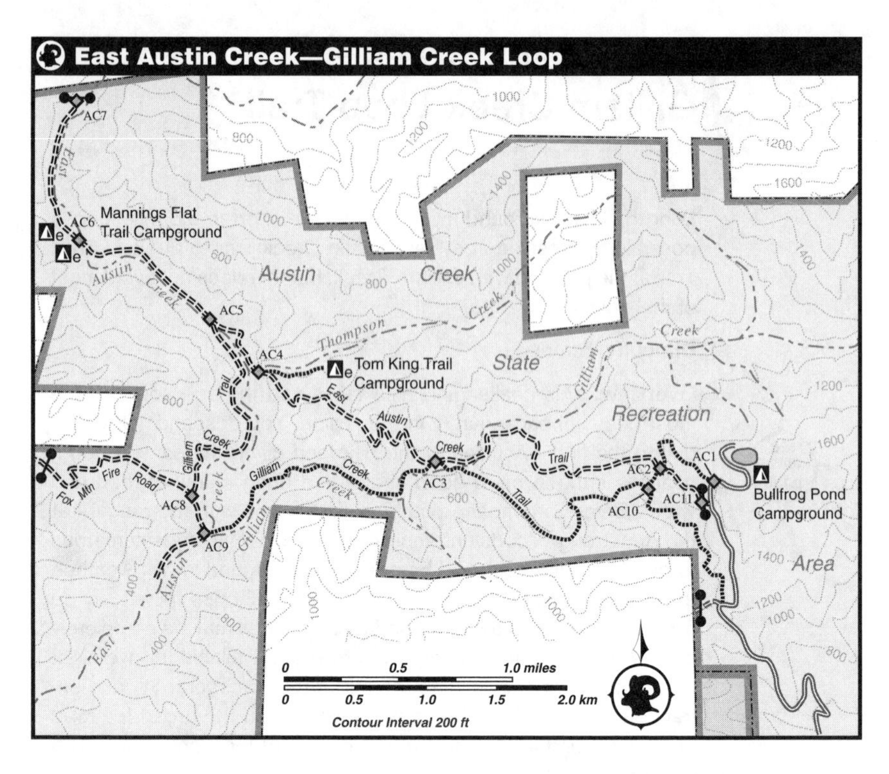

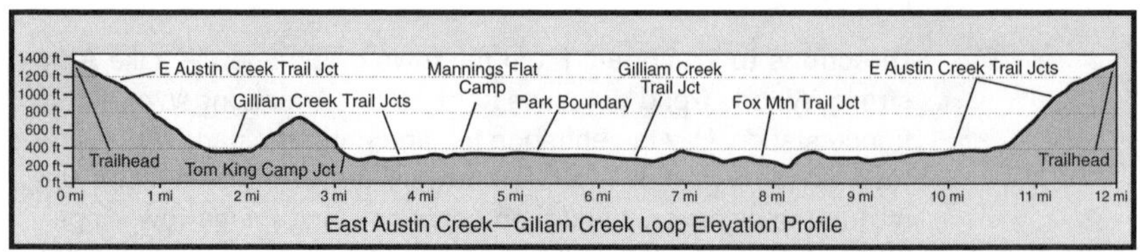

The trail alternates between open grasslands and shaded forests of oaks, madrones, bay trees, Douglas-firs, and manzanita. At 0.1 mile a side trail on your right leads to Bullfrog Campground. The trail curves sharply left at 0.3 mile and descends to join East Austin Creek Trail at 0.5 mile. Turn right and continue down this broad fire road. After 50 feet, notice a narrow single-track trail that descends steeply on your left. Remember this, as it will be your return route near the end of the loop.

East Austin Creek Trail descends through oak woodlands. Purists like to call this former county road by its original name, Panorama Grade. Look to the northwest as you hike. The reddish-colored vertical canyon on the distant ridge is Red Slide, site of a now-closed magnesite mine. Mule teams used to haul magnesite ore along your trail from Red

Slide to the railroad depot in Guerneville. When a 2-foot gauge railroad was built in the early 1900s the route was changed so the ore cars went to Magnesia Station south of Cazadero. There the ore was loaded onto narrow-gauge cars of the North Pacific Coast Railroad. Today the trail serves as a principal access route for Tom King Camp and Mannings Flat Camp.

The trail passes through a grove of oaks and levels briefly at 1.0 mile, then continues descending. You come to East Austin Creek at 1.4 miles and reach a concrete stock tank fed by a spring at 1.5 miles. Don't drink this water without first purifying it.

You near the bottom of the descent at 1.6 miles. At 1.8 miles you cross a wooden bridge over East Austin Creek and come to the junction with Gilliam Creek Trail, your first chance at an early return. If you return now along Gilliam Creek Trail, your total hike will be only 3.8 miles.

For this hike, keep right and continue along East Austin Creek Trail. You soon begin a 400-foot climb up the side of Morrison Ridge, reaching the summit at 2.7 miles and the junction with Tom King Camp on your right at 3.2 miles. This trail camp is an optional 0.5-mile round trip along the banks of Thompson Creek.

Along East Austin Creek Trail. (Photo by Lincoln Turner)

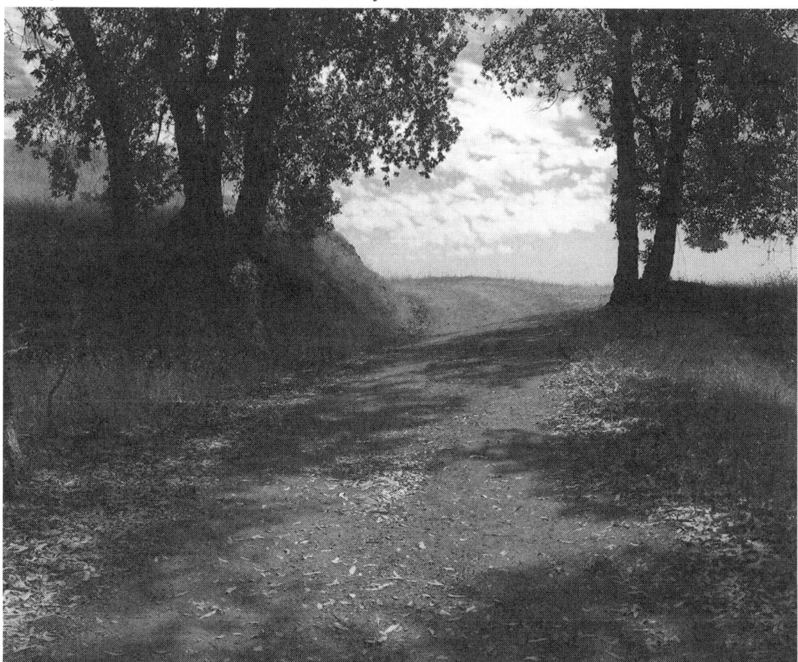

Continuing on, you cross a wooden bridge over Thompson Creek where it empties into East Austin Creek at 3.3 miles. Your trail is now heading northwest alongside East Austin Creek. At 3.7 miles you reach a second junction with Gilliam Creek Trail on the left. You will take this junction on your return trip, but for now, continue along East Austin Creek Trail toward Mannings Flat Trail Camp. At 4.0 miles, an old metal cage used to capture wild pigs sits in the shade of a tree on your left. Although efforts are being made to remove these descendents of escaped domestic pioneer livestock, you are still likely to see a herd or two at some point along your hike.

You ford East Austin Creek and enter Mannings Flat Trail Camp at 4.5 miles. In the dry season you can usually rock-hop across the creek without getting wet, but after seasonal rains it may be impassible.

First up is Lower Mannings Flat, with campsites along the creek. A few hundred yards farther, you reach Upper Mannings Flat. The campsites include picnic tables and metal fire rings, but check with rangers before making a fire. During the dry season, all open flame may be prohibited.

If you choose to return at this point, you can deduct 1.7 miles from the total trip. If you're still energetic, continue along a fairly level trail to a locked gate at the park boundary at 5.2 miles.

It is now time to make the long trek back. Return through Mannings Flat Camp and back to the junction with Gilliam Creek Trail at 6.7 miles. Turn right onto Gilliam Creek Trail and ford the creek. You may need to do a little exploring to find a suitable crossing.

Your trail now climbs beside the creek through a forest of firs and bay trees to a summit at 7.0 miles. As you descend past the summit, you reach the junction with Fox Mountain Trail on the right at 7.9 miles. Keep left here and continue your descent through mixed forest and open grassland.

Gilliam Creek Trail departs on the left from the fire road at 8.2 miles, becoming a single-track path for the remainder of the way. It quickly crosses East Austin Creek, wet during most of the year. A picnic bench just across the creek is a convenient place to take a break. This was once the location of Gilliam Creek Trail Camp, but it is now closed because of severe fire danger and is not expected to reopen.

You begin a sharp climb through dense woods at 8.6 miles. Poison oak abounds along this stretch, so be extra alert along here. Over the next couple of miles the trail crosses Gilliam Creek numerous times. Most of the crossings are well marked with wooden signs or rock cairns.

Your trail continues through mixed forest all the way to a junction with East Austin Creek Trail at 10.1 miles. You could choose to cross the creek here and return the way you came, but I recommend staying on the more shaded Gilliam Creek Trail for the upcoming steep climb back to the trailhead.

After the junction, Gilliam Creek Trail leaves its namesake creek and climbs alongside Schoolhouse Creek toward Gilliam Ridge. The trail climbs steeply for the remainder of the hike—in the next 1.8 miles you gain 800 feet of elevation. Just as you emerge from a stand of oaks at 11.3 miles you reach a junction with an unsigned single-track trail on your left that climbs sharply uphill. This is the short side trail to East Austin Creek Trail you saw on your way down. While you could keep right and stay on Gilliam Creek Trail, you can save more than a mile by taking this side trail over to East Austin Creek Trail. It connects just west of the junction with Vista Point Trail, your original route. Take Vista Point Trail and return along your original route to your car at 11.9 miles.

Trail 23: Austin Creek–Gilliam Creek Loop Trail Waypoints (WGS84 Datum)

Name	Latitude	Longitude	Feature
AC1	N38° 33.849′	W123° 00.754′	Vista Trail trailhead at parking area
AC2	N38° 33.881′	W123° 00.977′	Vista Trail junction with East Austin Creek Trail
AC3	N38° 33.909′	W123° 02.118′	Connector from East Austin Creek Trail to Gilliam Creek Trail
AC4	N38° 34.216′	W123° 02.880′	Tom King Camp trail junction
AC5	N38° 34.441′	W123° 03.223′	Junction of East Austin Creek Trail and Gilliam Creek Trail
AC6	N38° 34.722′	W123° 03.835′	Mannings Flat Campground
AC7	N38° 35.248′	W123° 03.853′	End of East Austin Creek Trail
AC8	N38° 33.830′	W123° 03.277′	Junction of Gilliam Creek Trail and Fox Mountain Trail
AC9	N38° 33.662′	W123° 03.230′	Gilliam Creek Trail departs on the east from the fire road
AC10	N38° 33.818′	W123° 01.052′	Junction with connector trail to East Austin Creek Trail
AC11	N38° 33.741′	W123° 00.742′	East Austin Creek trailhead at Armstrong Woods Road

Trail 24: East Ridge-McCray Ridge Loop Trail

Length: 2.1 miles round trip, 1.3 hours

Difficulty: Moderate

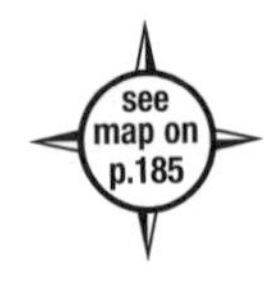

Overview: Enjoy the solitude and marvel at the scenery as you hike this little-used loop trail around the western flank of McCray Mountain. For most of its length you climb a wide, easily traveled fire road. At the top of the hike, a short stretch of single-track trail winds through open forest with moderate undergrowth before joining another fire road for the descent back to your car. At several points along the way you have magnificent views south and west all the way to Santa Rosa and beyond.

Directions to Trailhead: Same as Trail 23.

Trail Description. From the parking area, walk east along Armstrong Woods Road toward the campground. After 200 feet, you reach the East Ridge trailhead on your right. Take this trail and begin a steady climb along a broad fire road. You quickly reach an iron gate that blocks automobile traffic. Go around it and continue your climb through a mixed forest of redwoods, bay trees, California hazel, tanoaks, sword ferns, and wild roses. At 0.2 mile you reach a junction where a service road on your right leads to a large wooden water tank. If you look carefully in the woods just to the right of the service road you'll spot an ancient wooden birdhouse nailed to a tree, a leftover remnant from when this was private land prior to 1964.

Stay on the main trail, which soon curves right and continues uphill. You reach the junction with McCray Ridge Trail on your left at 0.2 mile. You will return via this trail, but for now, keep right and continue your climb. You emerge from the forest at 0.3 mile and soon come to the junction with a narrow footpath on your right. Take a short side trip along this path for a few hundred feet to a point with outstanding views to the south and west. Although the footpath continues on down the side of the mountain, return back to the junction at 0.4 mile and continue along the fire road. The trail levels briefly and then resumes climbing as it winds through alternating stretches of open forest and grassland. You pass a trailer and antenna tower used for State Parks communications at 0.5 mile.

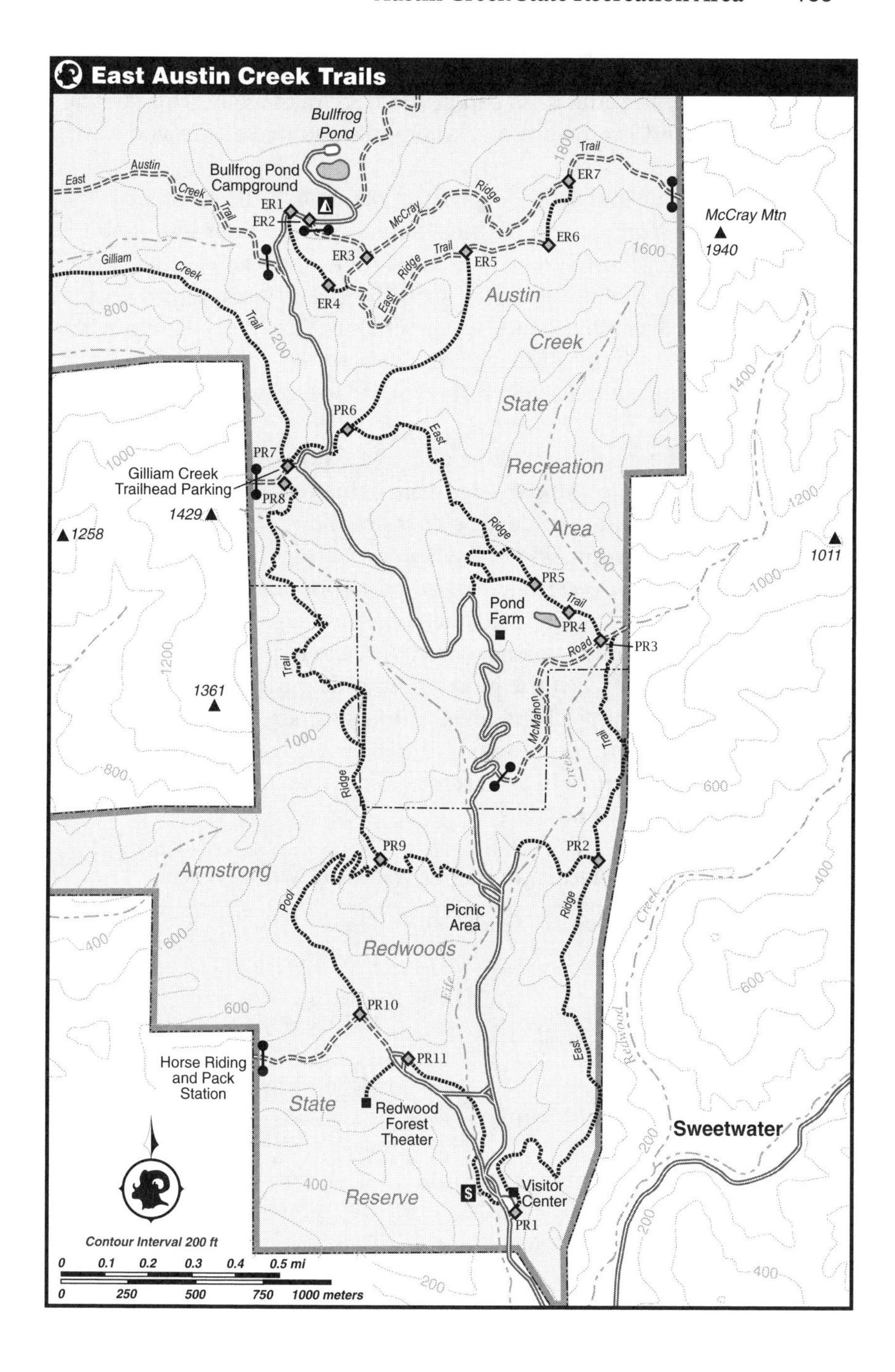
East Austin Creek Trails
Bullfrog Pond
Bullfrog Pond Campground
East Austin Creek Trail
McCray Ridge Trail
East Ridge Trail
Gilliam Creek Trail
McCray Mtn
1940
Austin Creek State Recreation Area
ER1
ER2
ER3
ER4
ER5
ER6
ER7
PR1
PR2
PR3
PR4
PR5
PR6
PR7
PR8
PR9
PR10
PR11
Gilliam Creek Trailhead Parking
1429
1258
1361
1011
East Ridge Trail
Pond Farm
Pond Farm Trail
McMahon Road
Ridge Trail
Pool Ridge Trail
Fife Creek
Redwood Creek
Armstrong Redwoods State Reserve
Picnic Area
Horse Riding and Pack Station
Redwood Forest Theater
Visitor Center
Sweetwater
Contour Interval 200 ft
0 0.1 0.2 0.3 0.4 0.5 mi
0 250 500 750 1000 meters

The forest ends at 0.6 mile, and you have more great views far southwest all the way to Santa Rosa and beyond, 25 miles away. This stretch of open grassland can be hot on a sunny day, so make sure you have plenty of water.

The trail levels and then descends at 0.9 mile, but resumes climbing by 1.0 mile. You pass an old steel animal trap on your left, used to capture wild pigs. The fire road ends at 1.1 miles and a single-track footpath heads north. Follow this faint path through a forest of redwoods and manzanita to reach another steel animal trap and the junction with McCray Ridge Trail at 1.3 miles. Turn left here and follow this eroded fire road through mixed forest as it descends southwest back toward the trailhead.

For the remainder of your hike along McCray Ridge Trail, you are in the shaded forest of tanoaks, redwoods, madrone, and bay trees, a welcome relief on a warm day. Be cautious along this stretch, as the trail is covered with tanoak and bay leaves that can be slippery in wet weather. At 1.8 miles, you reach old state park boundary signposts. This is no longer accurate, as recent acquisitions have expanded these limits. Today, your entire hike remains within the current park boundaries.

At 1.9 miles you reach the junction with East Ridge Trail that you saw near the beginning of the hike. Turn right here and retrace your steps downhill. As you descend, you can hear the sounds of the campground below on your right. You return to the road at 2.0 miles and are back at your car by 2.1 miles.

Trails 24–25: East Ridge–McCray Ridge Trail Waypoints (WGS84 Datum)

Name	Latitude	Longitude	Feature
ER1	N38° 33.855′	W123° 00.732′	Parking area
ER2	N38° 33.838′	W123° 00.686′	Junction of Road and East Ridge Trail
ER3	N38° 33.768′	W123° 00.541′	Junction of East Ridge and McCray Ridge Trails
ER4	N38° 33.711′	W123° 00.638′	Viewpoint on side trail–outstanding views to south and west
ER5	N38° 33.780′	W123° 00.285′	Junction of fire road and East Ridge Trail to ranger station
ER6	N38° 33.790′	W123° 00.078′	End of fire road. Single track trail heads north.
ER7	N38° 33.910′	W123° 00.025′	Junction of single track trail and McCray Ridge Trail

Trail 25: East Ridge-Pool Ridge Loop

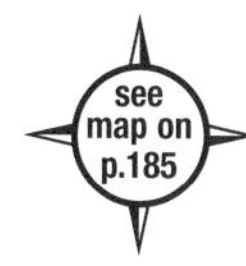

Length: 6.0 miles round trip, 3.5 hours

Difficulty: Strenuous

Overview: This challenging hike starts and ends in redwood forest, while the center portion traverses wooded grasslands. For the first 3 miles you climb a total of 1200 feet through sheltered forest along East Ridge Trail. The initial 500 feet of your climb lies within Armstrong Redwoods and the remainder within Austin Creek. At the top, you take Gilliam Creek Trail just long enough to cross over to Pool Ridge Trail for the descent. You have several chances for an early return along the way, but even the shortest loop involves considerable elevation gain. This loop is suitable for equestrians as well as hikers.

Directions to Trailhead: From the town of Guerneville, take Armstrong Woods Road 2.4 miles north to the Armstrong Woods entrance station. The visitor center parking area is on your right just prior to the entrance station. Currently, this parking area is free of charge. If there is space, park here. Otherwise, park along Armstrong Woods Road. East Ridge trailhead is just southeast of the visitor center, adjacent to the restrooms.

Trail Description. Before starting out on this hike, be sure you are prepared. Carry snacks and plenty of water. Check in at the visitor center for maps and information on current trail conditions.

From the trailhead, you immediately begin a steady climb through a forest of redwoods, bay trees, and tanoaks. Sword ferns and California hazel line the trailside. The trail curves right at 0.3 mile and for several hundred feet you walk along the tops of numerous tree roots. At various points along the way, trail crews have had to cut a path through fallen logs to maintain the trail.

You reach the crest of a local ridge at 0.4 mile and soon begin a brief descent. When you resume climbing at 0.6 mile, the redwoods are gone and the forest has changed to Douglas-fir, oak, and madrone. You have good views of the surrounding forest as you continue up and down through the wooded hills. You reach a Y-junction at 0.7 mile, but both trails quickly converge, so you can take either path. Just beyond lies a simple wooden bench where you might want to take a short break after your strenuous initial climb.

When ready, continue your ascent, being careful to avoid poison oak along the trail. You reach a crest at 1.0 mile, and then descend slightly to the junction with East Ridge Spur Trail at 1.2 miles. If you are ready to return, you can descend this steep, winding trail down to the picnic area and back along Pioneer Trail to the park entrance.

The described trail continues on through mixed forest. It stays fairly level for 0.2 mile, but a steep cliff looms on your left, so keep children under control along here. You resume climbing at 1.4 miles, briefly breaking out of the forest at 1.5 miles. You soon reenter a mixed forest of oaks, bay trees, Douglas-fir, and California buckeye.

You reach McMahon Road at 1.8 miles. Turn left here and cross a steel bridge. This service road eventually connects to Armstrong Woods Road and gives you a second chance for an early return. If you choose to walk back down narrow Armstrong Woods Road from here to the picnic area, be extremely cautious of oncoming vehicles.

East Ridge Trail continues uphill to the right just after the bridge. You come to Pond Farm's namesake pond at 1.9 miles, where a wooden bench honors Russ Whitman, a longtime park volunteer. Your trail levels briefly and then begins a steady climb. At 2.1 miles you pass a ranger's residence on the left and a gnarled oak with a hollow center resembling a goosepen. The trail here is lightly traveled, and you are likely to hear owls and woodpeckers as you continue your climb in solitude.

You break out of the forest and reach Horse Haven Meadow at 2.6 miles, complete with watering trough a short distance later. Bracken ferns grow profusely in the grassland along here. At 2.7 miles you reach a trail junction and the top of this hike, having climbed over 1200 feet from the parking lot far below. If you're not yet ready to return, you may want to continue on East Ridge Trail, which heads uphill on your right to the junction with McCray Ridge Trail and Bullfrog Pond Campground. For the described hike, though, turn left and take the Gilliam Creek Trail to begin your descent. Cross Armstrong Woods Road at 2.8 miles and continue down through mixed forest to the Gilliam Creek Trailhead parking area at 2.9 miles.

Don't take Gilliam Creek Trail, as it heads far away from your destination. Instead, follow the dirt fire road southwest a few hundred feet to another parking area and the Pool Ridge Trailhead on your left. Take this trail and begin a steep descent through open grassland, with great views southeast to Forestville and beyond. A series of wooden steps at 3.0 miles aids your descent just as you reenter the forest.

Your trail alternately climbs and descends as it snakes through the forest. At 3.4 miles you begin a sustained descent through a section of red clay soil that can be slippery when wet. Look for an outcrop of blueschist, a metamorphic rock, on your right at 3.6 miles, just after you cross a wooden bridge. You reach another trail junction at 3.9 miles. The main trail continues ahead, while the trail on the right loops over to an abandoned apple orchard before rejoining the main trail at 4.0 miles.

You briefly break out of the forest at 4.1 miles, but by 4.3 miles you have reentered the forest and reached a junction with a steep side trail on the left that leads down to the picnic area. Stay on Pool Ridge Trail, continuing downhill. You quickly reach a series of switchbacks that wind down the side of a forested ridge. At 4.8 miles you make the first of several crossings of a seasonal creek. The trail here may be impassible after recent rains. Watch for ancient redwood stumps, remnants of the logging era of the late 1800s. Several of these have mature second-growth fairy rings whose trunks are now more than 5 feet in diameter.

You pass under a fallen Douglas-fir at 5.1 miles and reach the junction with the road to the pack station at 5.2 miles. Turn left here and head down toward the Colonel Armstrong Tree parking area, which you reach at 5.3 miles. Walk over and admire the Colonel Armstrong Tree, then continue over to the Discovery Trail on your right. Walk down this trail, crossing the road twice, until you reach the ranger's kiosk and the park entrance at 5.9 miles. Return across the parking lot to your starting point, the East Ridge Trailhead, at 6.0 miles.

Trail 25: East Ridge-Pool Ridge Loop Trail Waypoints (WGS84 Datum)

Name	Latitude	Longitude	Feature
PR1	N38° 31.933′	W123° 00.150′	East Ridge Trail trailhead at Armstrong parking lot
PR2	N38° 32.613′	W122° 59.942′	Junction with trail descending steeply to picnic area
PR3	N38° 33.033′	W122° 59.933′	Junction with McMahon Road
PR4	N38° 33.085′	W123° 00.022′	Picnic bench overlooking pond at Pond Farm
PR5	N38° 33.138′	W123° 00.110′	Junction with trail back to Armstrong Woods Road
PR6	N38° 33.434′	W123° 00.588′	Junction of East Ridge Trail and Gilliam Creek Trail
PR7	N38° 33.369′	W123° 00.711′	Gilliam Creek trailhead parking area
PR8	N38° 33.336′	W123° 00.756′	Pool Ridge Trail departs downhill from fire road
PR9	N38° 32.608′	W123° 00.503′	Picnic table and junction with steep trail to picnic area
PR10	N38° 32.308′	W123° 00.543′	Junction with road to pack station
PR11	N38° 32.225′	W123° 00.427′	Junction with trail to picnic area

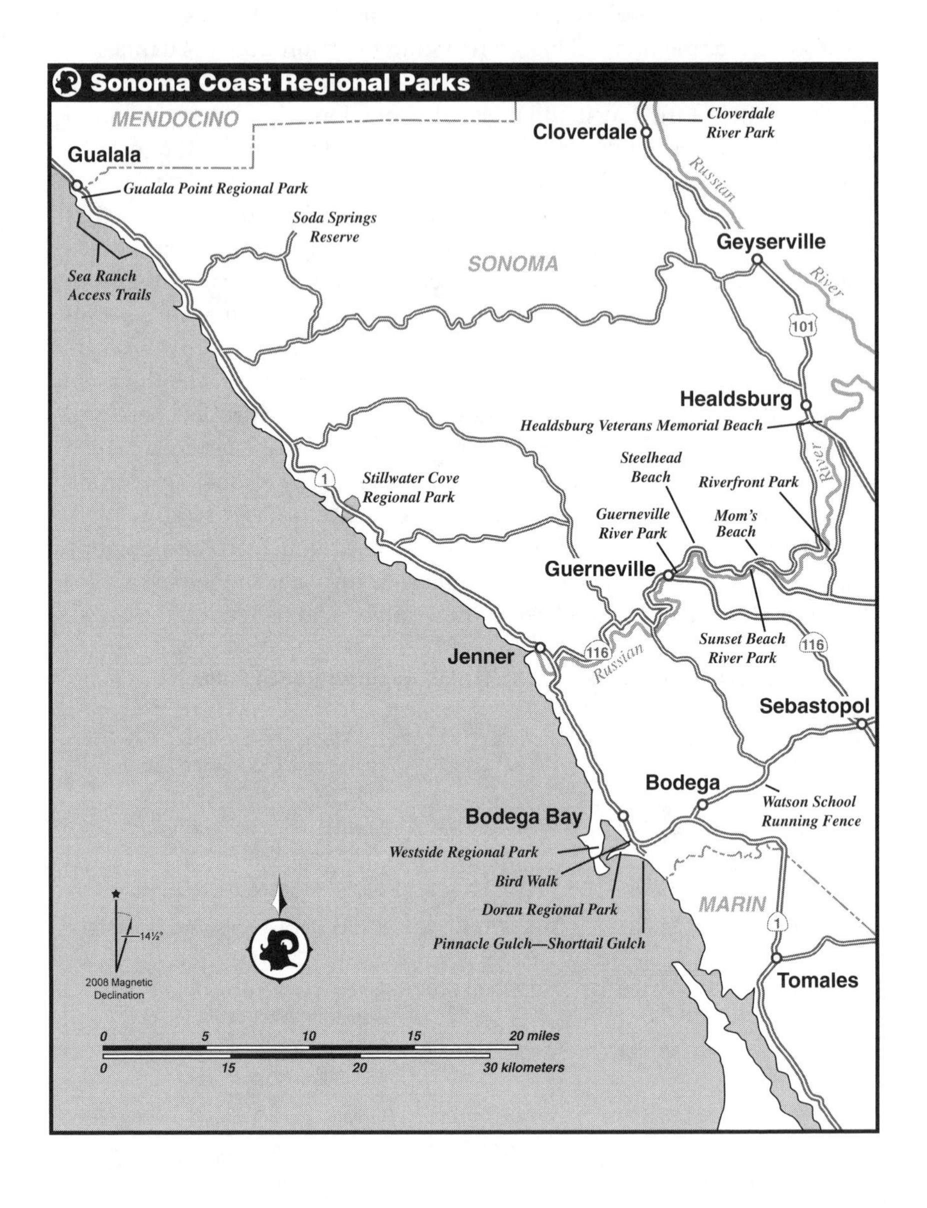
Sonoma Coast Regional Parks
MENDOCINO
Cloverdale
Cloverdale
River Park
Gualala
Gualala Point Regional Park
Russian
Soda Springs
Reserve
Geyserville
SONOMA
Sea Ranch
Access Trails
River
101
Healdsburg
Healdsburg Veterans Memorial Beach
Steelhead
Beach
Riverfront Park
River
1
Stillwater Cove
Regional Park
Guerneville
River Park
Mom's
Beach
Guerneville
Jenner
116
Russian
Sunset Beach
River Park
116
Sebastopol
Bodega
Watson School
Running Fence
Bodega Bay
Westside Regional Park
Bird Walk
Doran Regional Park
Pinnacle Gulch—Shorttail Gulch
MARIN
1
Tomales
14½°
2008 Magnetic
Declination
0
5
10
15
20 miles
0
15
20
30 kilometers

Chapter 7

Sonoma County Regional Parks

California's state parks aren't your only choices for recreational activities along the Sonoma Coast and Russian River. The County of Sonoma maintains a network of over 40 regional parks throughout the county, 16 of which lie near the coast or along the river. They offer a full range of recreational opportunities, including hiking, bicycling, picnicking, horseback riding, camping, fishing, swimming, canoeing, kayaking, and simply lying in the sun on a sandy beach.

If you're a dog lover, you'll also find the regional parks to be more dog-friendly than state parks. With only a few exceptions, dogs on leashes are permitted in all regional parks, including along the trails. Of course you are expected to clean up after your dog, not only to keep the trails clean but also to prevent foxes, otters, raccoons, and other animals from becoming infected with potentially fatal diseases often found in canine waste.

This chapter describes the regional parks found along the Sonoma Coast and Russian River. For a full listing of all Sonoma County Regional Parks, visit their website at www.sonoma-county.org/parks/index.htm.

Regional Parks of the Sonoma Coast

Doran Park

Doran Park at the south end of Bodega Bay is one of the most popular regional parks. Its prime attraction is a 2-mile stretch of sandy beach where you can fly kites, build sand castles, take an extended walk along the shoreline, go fishing, surfing, or, on hot days, even swimming. The beach is reasonably sheltered, so it doesn't usually get the strong waves you often see on the northern beaches. As always along the northern coast, though, pay attention to the rules of ocean safety on Page 18.

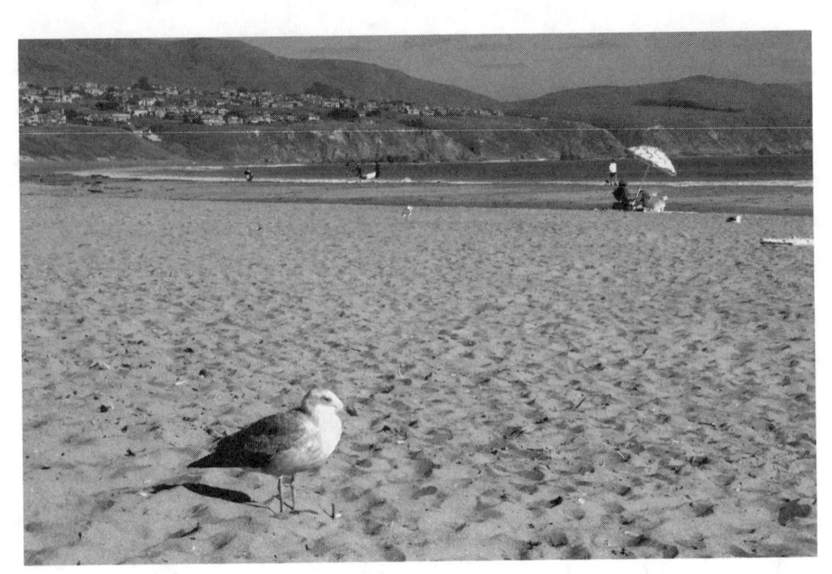

Doran Park.

Doran Park also has a popular campground that is open all year. With 134 sites, it's the largest of the regional parks campgrounds. Twenty sites are first-come-first-serve and 112 sites can be reserved in advance. There is also one group campsite and one site for hikers/bikers. Reservations must be made at least 10 days before your planned visit. You can reserve up to two campsites per party by calling 707-565-2267 or by going online at http://camping.sonoma-county.org/. The campsites lie on the exposed sand spit at the southern end of the harbor. A nearby foghorn sounds every 10 seconds day and night, so this may be a better spot for trailer and RV camping than for tent camping. Note, however, that there are no RV hookups at any of the campsites. The park's other facilities include a boat launch, dump station, fish cleaning station, picnic areas, restrooms with flush toilets, and pay-per-use showers.

Directions: From Santa Rosa, take Highway 12 to Sebastopol. As you cross Highway 116 at the town center, Highway 12 terminates and the road becomes Bodega Highway. Follow it all the way to its end at the junction with Highway 1. Turn right and follow Highway 1 north through Cheney Gulch for just over 3 miles. Just as you get to the outskirts of Bodega Bay, turn left onto Doran Park Road. Keep left onto Doran Beach Road for a half mile to the park entrance. An entry fee is charged for vehicles.

Bird Walk

Bodega Bay is one of the top sites for bird watching in North America, and the Bird Walk is an ideal location for viewing the numerous species that stop over on their winter migrations. A paved, disabled-accessible trail loops around a restored saltwater marsh at the southeast end of the bay. The park is open sunrise to sunset all year, and includes a paved parking area, picnic tables, and a chemical toilet. A fee is charged for parking.

Migratory birds spend summers in more northerly climates, so the months of May through July have the fewest birds here. The birds begin arriving on their southerly migration in late August and continue through October. By November, they have settled in for the winter. The northern migration begins as early as February for some species and continues through April. To learn more about birding in Sonoma County, visit the Madrone Audubon Society website at http://audubon.sonoma.net.

In late 2008, Sonoma County, in partnership with the Coastal Conservancy, opened a new trail that connects Bird Walk to Doran Beach. This trail includes a $500,000 bridge across Cheney Creek and is the first step in what will eventually be a 3-mile path through Bodega Bay to Salmon Creek.

Directions: From Santa Rosa, take Highway 12 to Sebastopol. As you cross Highway 116 at the town center, Highway 12 terminates and the road becomes Bodega Highway. Follow it all the way to its end at the junction with Highway 1. Turn right and follow Highway 1 north through Cheney Gulch for just over 3.5 miles. The Bird Walk parking area is on your left just beyond North Harbor Drive, on the south side of Bodega Bay. GPS coordinates for the trailhead are: N38° 19.216′ W123° 02.102′.

Pinnacle Gulch/Shorttail Gulch Coastal Access Trail

Pinnacle Gulch Trail is a steep, half-mile-long dirt path through coastal scrub that leads down to a secluded, sandy beach on the south side of Bodega Bay. The trailhead and a small parking area with restrooms are on Mockingbird Lane in the Bodega Harbour subdivision.

Nearby Shorttail Gulch Trail, opened in 2004, is the first new coastal access trail in the region since the 1980s. It departs from Osprey Drive, but there is no parking at this trailhead, so hikers must park at the Pinnacle Gulch parking lot and walk a half mile to the trailhead. From there, it's another half-mile hike and a 200-foot descent to a secluded beach. Watch for poison oak along either trail.

The beach at Shorttail Gulch is separated from Pinnacle Gulch to the north by two rocky points with a third beach in between. It is possible to cross these rocky points at low tide, so with care, athletic hikers can make a loop hike down Shorttail Gulch Trail, cross over to the beach at Pinnacle Gulch, and back up Pinnacle Gulch Trail to the parking lot. Total round-trip distance for this hike is almost exactly 2 miles.

Directions: From Santa Rosa, take Highway 12 to Sebastopol. As you cross Highway 116 at the town center, Highway 12 terminates and the road becomes Bodega Highway. Follow it all the way to its end at the junction with Highway 1. Turn right and follow Highway 1 north through Cheney Gulch for just over 3 miles. Just as you get to the outskirts of Bodega Bay, turn left onto Harbor Way, then left again onto Heron Drive. Drive 0.9 mile and turn left onto to Mockingbird Drive. The Pinnacle Gulch parking area is 0.1 mile down Mockingbird Drive. GPS coordinates for the trailhead at Pinnacle Gulch are N38°18.772′ W123°00.842′ and for the trailhead at Shorttail Gulch are N38°18.519′ W123°00.689′.

Westside Park

This park sits along the flat shores of Bodega Bay and is oriented toward fishing. It essentially consists of a campground with 38 reservable sites and seven more first-come-first-served sites. There are no RV hookups, but the park includes flush toilets, showers, an RV dump station, a boat ramp, and a fish-cleaning station. A grocery store and tackle shop are nearby on Westshore Road. Fees are charged for both camping and day-use parking. Although the park doesn't include any hiking trails, Westside Trail (Trail 4) at Sonoma Coast State Park is just across the road. From there you have access to the full system of trails in Bodega Dunes.

Directions: From Santa Rosa, take Highway 12 to Sebastopol. As you cross Highway 116 at the town center, Highway 12 terminates and the road becomes Bodega Highway. Follow it all the way to its end at the junction with Highway 1. Turn right (north) and continue along Highway 1 through the town of Bodega Bay. At the north side of the town, turn left onto Eastshore Road, go down the hill, and turn right at the stop sign. This is Bay Flat Road, which becomes Westshore Road after about 0.2 mile. Westside Park is on your left 1.6 miles past the stop sign. GPS coordinates for the park are N38° 19.359′ W123° 03.365′.

Stillwater Cove

The prime attraction at 210-acre Stillwater Cove is abalone diving, but you can also enjoy a picnic with great ocean views or take a hike through a redwood forest. The Stillwater Cove campground has 22 sites, restrooms with flush toilets, pay-per-use showers, and an RV dump station (but no RV hookups). The cove is across the highway from the campground and day-use area. A launch facility at the cove is suitable for kayaks and small boats. There is no parking at the cove, so you must unload your equipment, then park at the day-use area or in any of the unmarked dirt pullouts along the road. There is a parking fee at the day-use area.

Canyon Loop Trail. This trail departs from the northwest end of the day-use parking lot and descends to Stockhoff Creek. When you reach the creek, a trail on your left goes to Stillwater Cove, while another goes across a wooden bridge over the creek. This will be your return path, but for now, keep right and take a third trail that stays on the near side of the creek. This trail winds through a second-growth redwood forest with a carpet of sword ferns and redwood sorrel. Notice the many fairy rings growing around central stumps. These secondary growths are now mature trees, indicating that this forest was logged many years ago. The trail eventually reaches a junction with a short side trail to the old Fort Ross Schoolhouse. This historic one-room school was opened at Fort Ross in 1885 and was moved several times before ending up at its present location in 1974. After departing the school, the trail loops back to the parking lot after a 1.2-mile hike.

Directions: From the town of Jenner, take Highway 1 north for 15 miles. The entrance to the Stillwater Cove campground and day-use area is on your right, 4 miles past Fort Ross. The turn-off for the beach launch is 0.1 mile farther on the left. GPS coordinates for the Canyon Loop Trailhead are N38° 32.853´ W123° 17.753´, and for the Fort Ross School are N38° 32.959´ W123° 17.683´.

Soda Springs Reserve

This quiet redwood grove in a remote corner of the county has been used as a park for over 100 years. It was originally a private campground operated by the Stibl family, who homesteaded the site beginning in the 1880s. Although the land was sold to the Wheeler Timber Company in 1910, the Stibl family continued as caretakers for the campground.

Wheeler Timber sold the park and surrounding lands to the Paul B. Kelly family in 1949. After her husband's death in 1955, Mrs. Kelly dedicated the park in his memory to the town of Annapolis. She improved the site with picnic tables and stone fireplaces.

The land changed hands several times over the next 30 years, and only after the Longview Fibre Company filed a timber harvest plan in 1985 was it discovered that Mrs. Kelly had never formally deeded the park to the town. The community quickly mobilized, and with help from the Save-the-Redwoods League and Coastal Forestlands, Ltd, they purchased and donated 49 acres to the County of Sonoma for a permanent park.

Sonoma County's Regional Parks allow dogs on most trails, including this one through a redwood tree at Soda Springs Reserve.

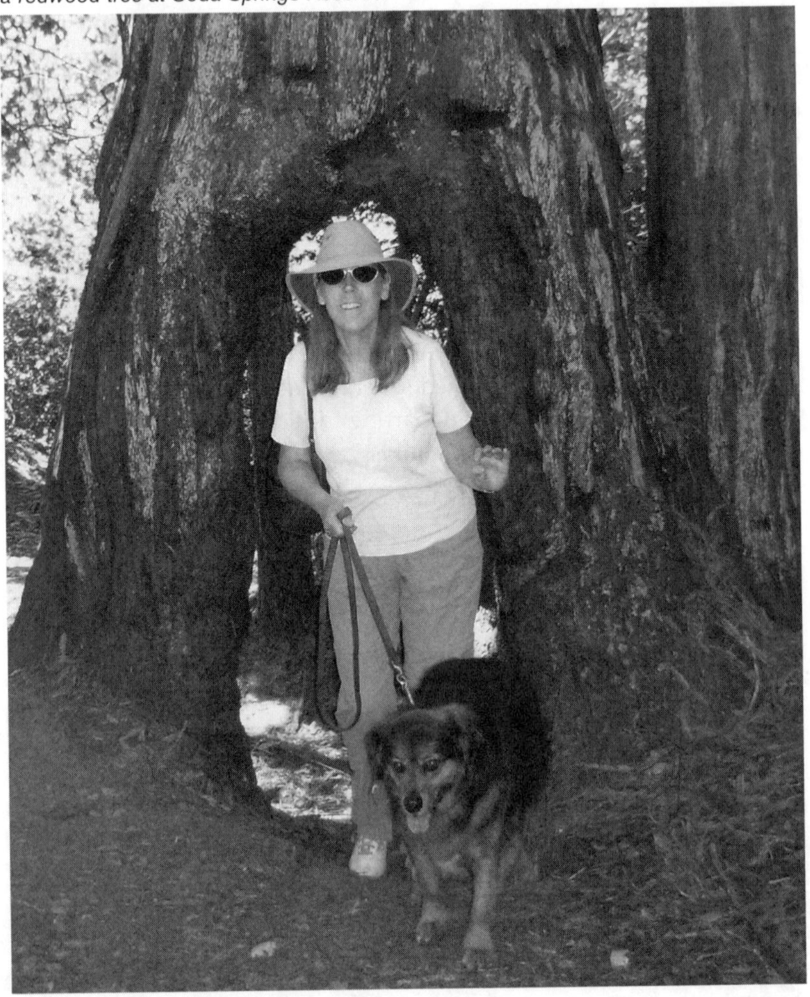

The park lies along Buckeye Creek, a tributary of the South Fork of the Gualala River. Although there are no major hiking trails, the park includes a picnic area with several parking spaces, three tables, stone fireplaces, and a cinderblock outhouse. Several short trails branch out from either side through the redwood forest, eventually ending at the creek. Poison oak grows profusely along these trails, so keep pets and children under control. Dog-friendly Buckeye Creek usually has shallow pools of water even in late summer, making it ideal for splashing on a hot day.

The park's remote location means you may be the only one there even on a summer weekend. There are no services after leaving Highway 1, so be sure to bring food and water with you. Soda Springs Reserve is one of the few regional parks that doesn't charge an admission fee.

Directions: The park lies 10.7 miles east of The Sea Ranch in northwest Sonoma County. From the town of Jenner, take Highway 1 north for 30 miles to the intersection with Annapolis Road. Turn right and follow Annapolis Road 7.5 miles to Soda Springs Road, passing through the hamlet of Annapolis along the way. Turn left at Soda Springs Road, which becomes Kelly Road after about 1.2 miles. This last stretch is on a well-maintained dirt road. The park is on your left 2.0 miles down Kelly Road. The route is well marked with signs at all intersections. GPS coordinates for the picnic area are: N38°44.717′ W123°20.954′

The Sea Ranch Access Trails

The land now known as The Sea Ranch was originally part of the German Rancho, a land grant given by the Mexican government to Ernest Rufus in 1846, only three months before California declared its independence. Under the new government, there was little interest in preserving the rights of the existing landowners. So the rancho was soon broken up and sold to a succession of owners over the years. By 1910, Walter Frick had purchased several parcels and formed the Rancho Del Mar. When Oceanic California, Inc., bought the land in 1963 to develop a unique coastal community, they translated the historic name into its English equivalent, The Sea Ranch.

Architect Al Boeke envisioned a community that would harmonize with the natural beauty of the land. Houses would be unpainted and no lawns or fences would be allowed. But part of the plan called for 10 miles of shoreline previously accessible to the public to be reserved only for residents. This concept met with stiff public resistance, resulting in years of legal battles. It was even directly responsible for the creation of the California Coastal Commission, an agency chartered with the responsibility to protect the State's coastal resources. The matter was not resolved until 1980, when the State legislature passed a bill permitting the development to continue on condition that easements be included for public access to the coast. As a result, there are now five access points along Highway 1 plus an extended trail along the bluffs.

The public trails are open from sunrise to sunset daily. Fees are charged at all parking lots, and rangers are diligent about ticketing vehicles that don't have a receipt. Recreational vehicles and vehicles with trailers are not allowed in the parking lots. Dogs on leashes are allowed on all trails, but bicycles are not. Fires are not permitted on the beaches.

Blufftop Trail. This 3-mile long trail runs from Gualala Point Regional Park south to the junction with Walk-On Beach Trail in The Sea Ranch. Until 2004, Blufftop Trail extended a few hundred feet farther south to Walk-On Beach. But in that year, a portion of the bluff collapsed, taking part of the trail with it. Although it would be easy enough to walk around the eroded stretch, the public easement does not extend the few extra feet necessary to make this possible. The county has been studying various options, but as this book goes to press, has not made any decisions. Until that happens, Walk-On Beach is closed to public access. Residents and visitors who are staying at The Sea Ranch can walk all the way to the beach.

Blufftop Trail's north trailhead at Gualala Point Regional Park is a dirt path that takes off from the paved trail south of the visitor center. GPS coordinates for this trailhead are: N38° 45.550′ W123° 31.439′.

Walk-On Beach Trail. This is the northernmost of five public access points along Highway 1 in The Sea Ranch. Please note that until the eroded portion of Blufftop Trail is repaired, you can't actually get to Walk-On Beach. However, the trail still serves as the southern access to Blufftop Trail. A small parking lot and outhouse at the trailhead sit on the west side of Highway 1 near milepost 56.50. GPS coordinates for the trailhead are: N38° 44.401′ W 123° 29.503′

Shell Beach Trail. This is the next public access point south of Walk-On Beach Trail. A half-mile-long trail leads to a sandy beach. The parking lot is at milepost 55.2. It has room for five to six cars and includes an outhouse at the trailhead. GPS coordinates are: N38° 43.745′ W123° 28.353′.

Stengel Beach Trail. This access point has the largest parking lot, with room for a dozen cars. Turn west from the highway near milepost 53.96 and into the parking lot. From here, it's a quarter-mile hike to Stengel Beach. GPS coordinates for the trailhead are: N38° 43.002´ W123° 27.479´.

Pebble Beach Trail. It is just over a quarter mile from this trailhead to a rocky beach. A small parking lot at milepost 52.3 includes an outhouse. GPS coordinates for the trailhead are: N38° 41.965´ W123°26.179´.

Black Point Beach Trail. This is the southernmost of the public access points. A quarter-mile-long path leads steeply down a staircase to a rocky beach at the north side of Black Point. The parking lot and outhouse are near milepost 50.83, at GPS coordinates N38°40.927´ W123°25.730´.

Gualala Point

This strikingly beautiful 195-acre park at the north end of the Sonoma Coast lies just south of the town of Gualala (pronounced wa-LA-la). The name comes from a Pomo Indian word meaning, "where the water flows down." It's an apt name for the place where the Gualala River empties into the Pacific Ocean. Besides day hiking and picnicking, it is also a popular spot for small weddings.

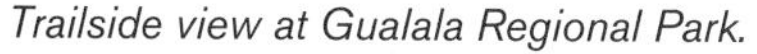

Trailside view at Gualala Regional Park.

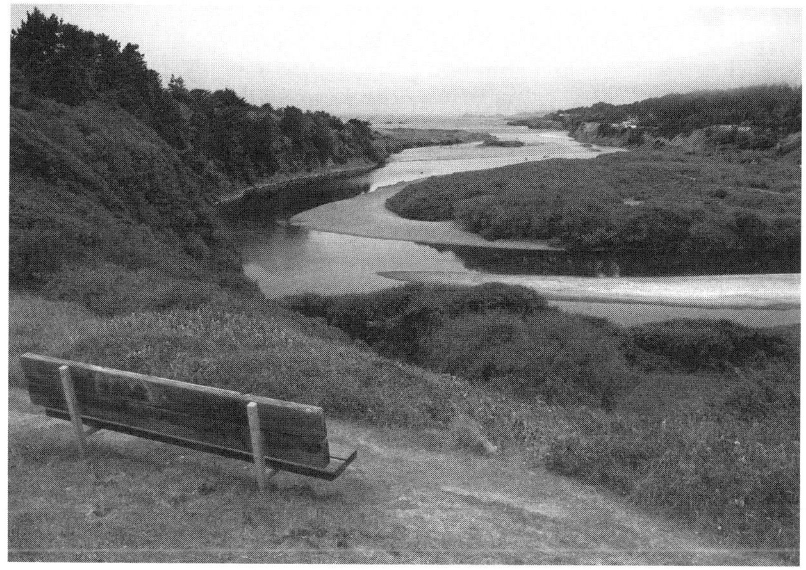

Several trails branch out from near the visitor center across the headlands. Take the paved trail at the south end of the visitor center parking lot for a half-mile trek down to the beach (GPS coordinates for the trailhead are N38° 45.508′ W123°31.384′). This is also the way to the trailhead for Blufftop Trail (see Page 198), which heads out on your left a few hundred feet down the path.

The park includes a visitor center, picnic area, and a 25-site campground in a redwood forest. Facilities include pay-per-use showers, restrooms with flush toilets, and a dump station for recreational vehicles. There are no RV hookups in the campsites.

Directions: The Park is on Highway 1 at the north end of Sonoma County. From the town of Jenner, drive 36 miles north. After passing through The Sea Ranch, you'll see the day-use and visitor center entrance on your left near milepost 58.20. The road to the campground is across the highway on the right.

Watson School/Running Fence

Watson School was built in 1856 to serve the children of local farmers and dairymen. It continued as a public school until 1967, longer than any other one-room school in California. It is named for James Watson, a pioneer settler who donated the land and along with the rest of the community, helped with its construction. The school was built in the traditional style of the day, except for an unusual sloping floor that created amphitheater-style seating. It is maintained today in its original condition. The school building itself is in need of repairs and so is closed to the public, but you are welcome to enjoy a picnic on the grounds outside.

The picnic grounds also include a plaque commemorating the Running Fence, an ambitious temporary art project created by the artists Christo and Jeanne-Claude, which ran through Sonoma and Marin Counties in 1976. It took four years of preparation, including a 450-page environmental impact report, numerous public hearings, and negotiations with 59 ranchers whose property would be crossed by the fence, before construction could begin. The fence consisted of 24.5 miles of white nylon fabric, 18 feet high, which was suspended from steel cable supported by over 2,000 steel poles. Construction took six months, after which it remained in place for only two weeks in September of that year.

The artists envisioned the fence running all the way to the sea and disappearing into the water, but the California Coastal Commission refused to grant permission for this last stretch. Their somewhat dubious logic was that doing so would dilute their ability to prohibit permanent construction in the future. Undaunted, the artists extended the fence into the sea anyway, leaving it just long enough to document in photographs. Happily the transgression didn't set the feared precedent, and the subsequent reaction was overwhelmingly positive. The general agreement was that it was an important step in completing the artistic vision.

Afterward the fence was completely dismantled, and no trace remains today. The whole project was funded entirely by the artists through the sale of preparatory drawings, scale models, and original artwork.

Directions: From Santa Rosa, take Highway 12 west to Sebastopol. As you cross Highway 116 at the town center, the road becomes Bodega Highway. Follow it 7.8 miles to Watson School on your left. There is a free parking area in front of the school.

Regional Parks of the Russian River

Guerneville River Park

Only a small portion of the land along the Russian River in Sonoma County is publicly accessible. This park in the center of Guerneville was opened in 2007 to provide public beach access. Facilities include a 12-space parking lot, picnic area, and restrooms. Additional improvements are still in the planning stage, including an outdoor stage for community events.

Directions: The park lies across the river from the town of Guerneville. You can either park in town and walk the pedestrian bridge across the Russian River to the park or drive the highway bridge across the river and immediately turn left onto Drake Road. Circle under the bridge and turn right into the parking lot. The park is open sunrise to sunset. A fee is charged for parking.

Steelhead Beach

This park near Forestville is a popular access point for the Russian River. A large, 75-space parking lot lies well off River Road, with a boat launch and trailer turning area at the edge of the river. The road ends at Steelhead Beach, a nice sandy beach on the south side of the river. Two short trails roughly follow the river and combine to form a mile-long loop. This is a day-use area only, open from sunrise to sunset. A fee is charged for parking.

This stretch of river is a relative rarity along the lower Russian River because it has never been extensively developed. Except for the remains of an old gravel screening plant just northeast of the parking lot, the park retains its natural ecosystem. A forest of cottonwoods, big-leaf maple, California bay, and Oregon ash lines the river, with willows, blackberries, fennel, and an assortment of wildflowers forming the understory. Steelhead Beach is a nice place to frolic in the river, but be aware there are no lifeguards here and fires are not allowed on the sand. The beach is a good place to launch kayaks or canoes.

You can hike to secluded Children's Beach by walking from the parking lot to the Willow Trail trailhead on your left just south of the trailer turning area. This trail is a shaded dirt path through mixed forest and reaches Children's Beach in 0.4 mile. Just before reaching the beach, you come to a junction with Osprey Trail on your left. For your return, take Osprey Trail through the forest for a half mile back to its trailhead at the road. From there, turn right and walk 500 feet back to the parking lot for a total round trip of 1.2 miles. GPS coordinates for the Willow Trail trailhead are N38° 29.976´ W122° 54.019´, for Osprey Trail trailhead are N38° 29.932´ W122°54.031´, and for Children's Beach are N38° 30.182´ W122°54.336´.

Directions: From Santa Rosa, take Highway 101 north to the River Road exit. Turn left and follow River Road 8.5 miles west. The park entrance is on your right.

Riverfront Park

This park along the Russian River near Windsor is on the site of a former gravel quarry. It includes three former gravel pits that have been converted to recreational lakes. The property was purchased in 2002 and opened in 2005 through collaboration with the Sonoma County Water Agency and the Sonoma County Agricultural Preservation and Open Space District.

The park is being developed in several phases. During the initial phase, the northernmost lake, Lake McLaughlin, is closed to the public. Both Lake Wilson in the middle and Lake Benoist to the south are open for fishing and non-motorized boating (swimming is not allowed). The park also includes a large picnic area in a towering redwood grove adjacent to the parking lot, and over 2 miles of level trails suitable for

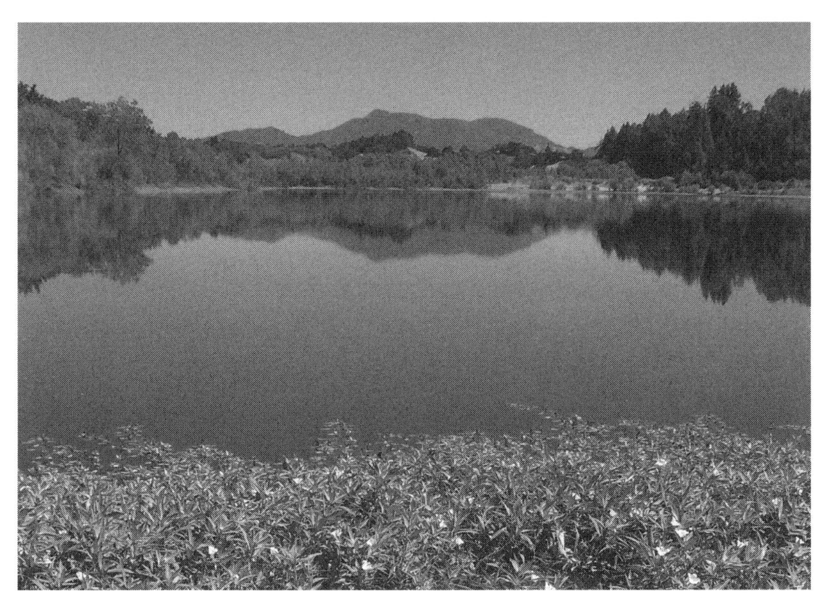

Mt. St. Helena is visible in this view looking across Lake Benoist at Riverfront Regional Park.

hikers, horseback riders, and mountain bikers. Another more strenuous trail winds 0.4 mile along a ridge through the redwood forest.

Lake Trail: This easy 2.3-mile hiking-biking-riding loop trail departs from the north side of the picnic area, along a good dirt road formerly used by gravel trucks. The broad, flat trail is ideal for novice mountain bikers or families with children. For the first 0.3 mile you head southwest, with the forested picnic area on your left and Lake Wilson behind a berm on your right.

When you reach Lake Benoist, keep to the right and follow the trail counterclockwise around the lake. Your trail, now in open sun, quickly passes several picnic tables with barbecue stands. Oaks, maples, walnuts, cottonwoods, and willows lie to your right, with the Russian River just beyond. Along the trail, fennel, blue elderberry, blackberries, and occasional poison oak lie closer to the ground.

Side trails branch off at several points, but stay on the broad dirt road and follow it around the lake. At 1.1 miles you come to a park bench with a great view across the water to distant Mount St. Helena. Continuing on, you briefly re-enter forest at 1.3 miles but are soon back in the sun. Cross a bridge over a concrete culvert at 1.7 miles and complete the loop around the lake at 1.9 miles.

From here, the easiest path is to retrace your steps back to the parking lot. But if you're up for a little more adventure, take the side trail that departs on your right into the forest at 2.0 miles. This is Redwood Hill Trail, a lightly traveled path through the forest that quickly climbs 100 feet up the side of a ridge. When you reach the top at 2.2 miles, keep left and begin descending down the back of the ridge. The sounds of traffic indicate you are now close to Eastside Road, but the trail soon makes a sweeping curve to the left, taking you away from the road and back toward the picnic area. Cross an iron bridge and enter the picnic area at 2.3 miles, and return to your car in the parking lot at 2.4 miles.

Directions: From Santa Rosa, take Highway 101 north to the River Road exit. Turn left and go west 5.4 miles along River Road to the junction with Trenton-Healdsburg Road. Turn right here and go north 1.3 miles to the intersection with Eastside Road. Keep right and follow Eastside Road 1.4 miles to the Riverfront Park entrance on the left. As you drive down the entrance road, you pass a dirt parking strip on the left for autos with horse trailers. The road turns sharply left after 0.1 mile and ends at a parking lot adjacent to the picnic area. GPS coordinates for the parking lot and trailhead are: N38° 31.116′ W122° 51.293′.

Forestville River Access/Mom's Beach

Mom's Beach has been a favorite spot for locals for a number of years. It was developed into a county park in response to public demand for greater access to the Russian River. Although by law Russian River beaches up to the "mean high water mark" are public lands, getting to them has not always been easy. The river is surrounded by private property, and landowners aren't appreciative of strangers tramping across their lands. This secluded access point leads to a nice beach just a short walk from the parking area. Get there early, as the beach tends to fill up fast on warm summer days.

Directions: From Santa Rosa, take Highway 101 north to the River Road exit. Turn left and go west about 10 miles. Just before you get to the Hacienda Bridge across the Russian River, you reach River Drive. Turn right, then quickly right again into the parking lot. From the parking lot, walk west along the road about 500 feet to a pathway between two houses leading to the beach. GPS coordinates for the trailhead are N38°30.586′ W122°55.419′.

Healdsburg Veterans Memorial Beach

Every year, the City of Healdsburg installs a summer dam on the Russian River to create a popular swimming area. This park is just upstream of the dam. It includes a large parking area, a broad, grassy picnic area with numerous tables and barbecue grilles, volleyball courts, a sandy beach, and restrooms with outdoor showers. Lifeguards are on duty during the season. Get there early, as this is such a popular park that it fills up fast on summer days. The dam is usually in place from Memorial Day through Labor Day, but dates vary depending on river conditions. To verify that the beach is open, call 707-433-1625.

Directions: From central Santa Rosa, take Highway 101 north for 13 miles to the Healdsburg Avenue exit and turn right. The park is on your left after a half mile. A fee is charged for parking.

Cloverdale River Park

This is the northernmost park along the Russian River in Sonoma County. It's a great spot for fishing, picnicking, or watching wildlife. A rustic picnic area along the river next to the parking lot includes tables with barbecues. You can also launch canoes or kayaks here, although there is no formal launching facility. A fee is charged for parking.

The trailhead for Makahmo Trail departs from the south end of the parking lot. This trail, named for the local Pomo Indians who once lived in the area, is a 1.1-mile (one-way) paved path along the river, ending on First Street in Cloverdale. Interpretive areas at various points along the way cover the natural and Native American history of the area. GPS coordinates for the trailhead are N38°49.353′ W123°00.644′.

Directions: From Santa Rosa, take Highway 101 north for 32 miles to the town of Cloverdale. At the north end of town, take the North Cloverdale/Highway 128 exit and turn right onto N. Redwood Highway. After 0.2 mile, turn right again onto McCray Road. The park is located 0.5 mile down McCray Road on the left.

Sunset Beach River Park

Sonoma County's newest regional park is Sunset Beach River Park on the Russian River, just west of Forestville. It was developed in partnership with the Sonoma County Agricultural and Open Space District, California State Parks, and the California Department of Boating and Waterways. Opened in July 2009, it provides public access to the river on a broad gravel bar at the edge of the water. Facilities include a paved parking lot with space for 30 vehicles (including 2 disabled accessible spaces), two portable restrooms adjacent to the parking lot, and four picnic tables at the edge of a shaded forest of black walnut, oak, and California bay trees. The gravel beach is a quarter-mile walk along a broad dirt road. Fires and barbecues are prohibited on the beach, but barbecues (bring your own) are permitted at the picnic tables. Dogs on leashes are welcome throughout the park. There are no boat launching facilities at this site, but you can carry kayaks or canoes to the beach.

View of Russian River and Hacienda Bridge from Sunset Beach.

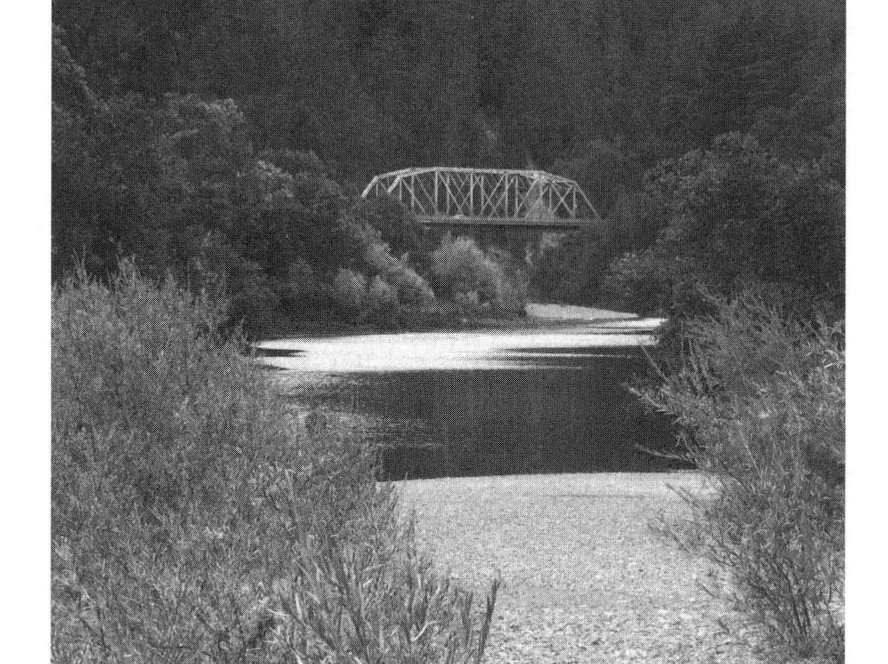

Directions: From Santa Rosa, take Highway 101 north to the River Road exit. Turn left and drive 10.9 miles west. After you cross the Hacienda Bridge (an iron truss bridge that originally carried railroad traffic), watch for the park entrance on your left. The park is open sunrise to sunset. A fee is charged for parking.

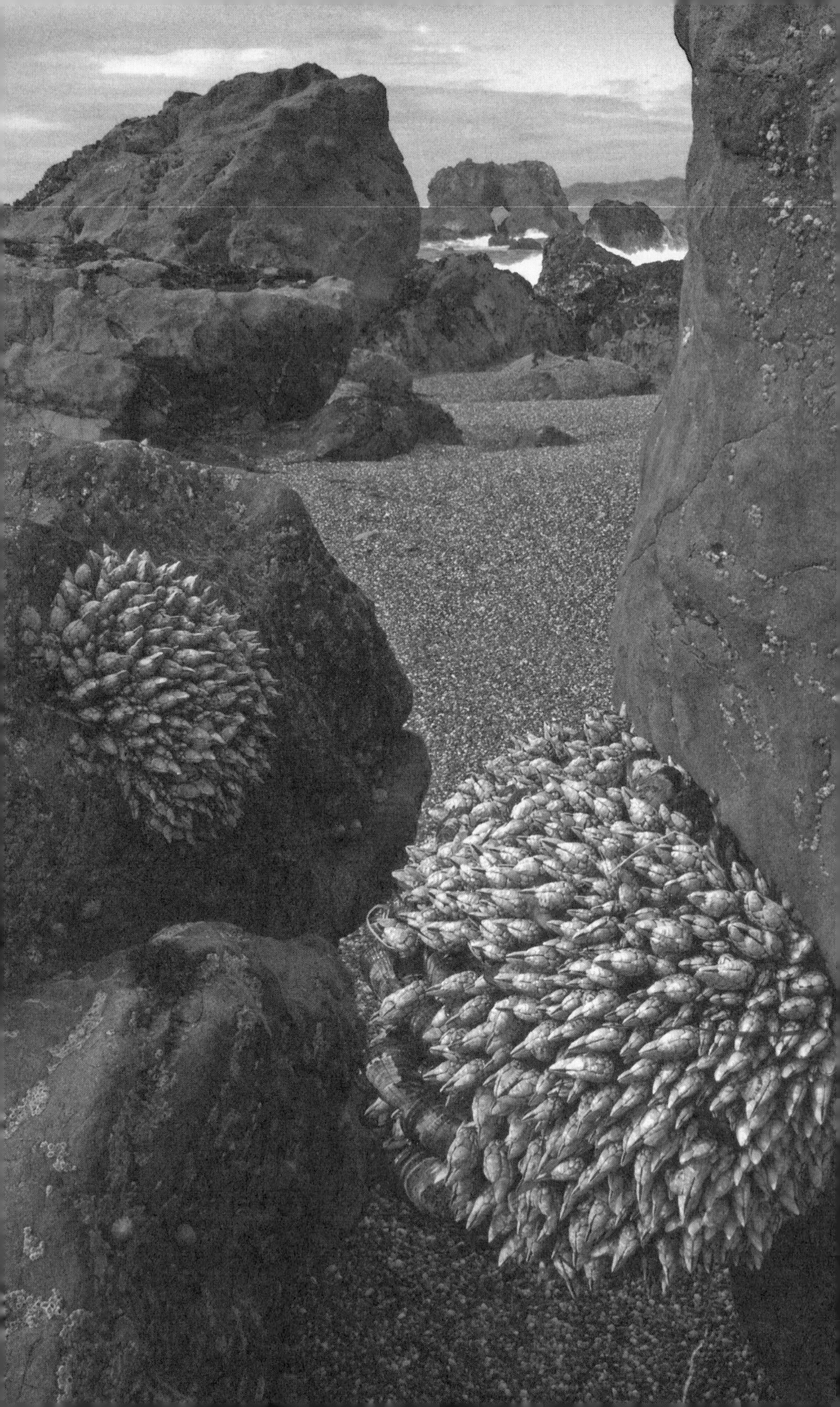

Appendix A

Common Tidepool Creatures of the Sonoma Coast

California Mussel

Mytilus californianus

Bluish-black shell to 10″ length. Often occurs in dense colonies on rocks exposed to surf, intermixed with barnacles. Mussels serve as food for numerous creatures, including sea stars, crabs, snails, birds, and sea otters. Also a favorite food for man.

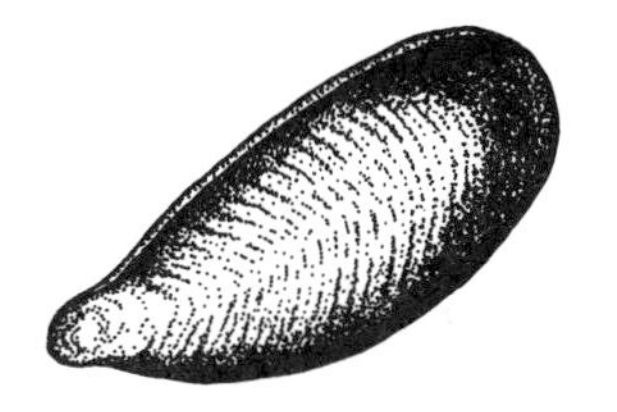

Caution: Mussels feed on a plankton from late May through October that causes them to be poisonous. Consult State fishing regulations for more information.

Red Abalone

Haliotis rufescens

Range from Alaska to central California. Found in rocky intertidal and subtidal areas to depths of as much as 300 feet. Shell to 12″ long by 9″ wide. Muscular foot can exert a strong grasp on rock, making them difficult to dislodge. Eat marine algae, especially various kelps. Besides man, chief predator is the sea otter. Related Black Abalone is slightly smaller.

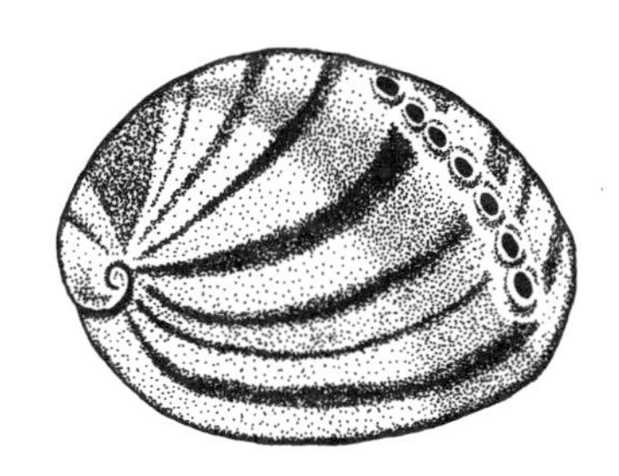

Left: *Leaf barnacles at Arched Rock Beach.*

Plate Limpet

Notoacmaea scutum

Oval, cone-shaped, brownish to greenish shell up to 1″ length. Limpets are related to abalones.

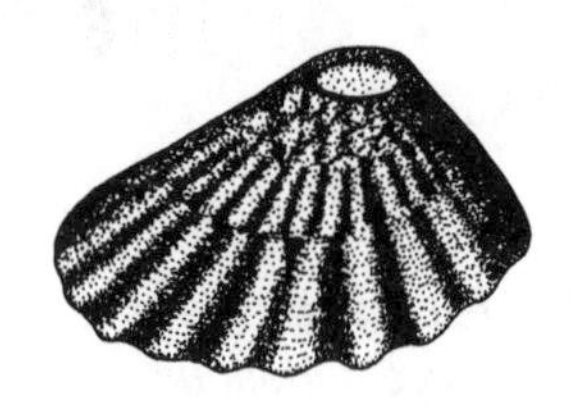

They have only a single shell, unlike clams, oysters, or mussels. They are found on rocks and in mussel beds between high and low tide lines. They feed on various algae and move only when wetted by waves or when they are under water. Related species include Ribbed Limpet, Rough Limpet, Shield Limpet, Owl Limpet, Dunce Cap Limpet, and Keyhole Limpet.

Black Katy Chiton

Katharina tunicata

Found on rocks exposed to heavy surf and full sun. Lengths to 5″. Chitons are mollusks related to abalone and mussels, and like other mollusks, they eat seaweed. Most species have eight overlapping plates on their backs. On the Black Katy Chiton, the plates are partially covered by a thick black girdle. Related species: Mossy Chiton, Lined Chiton, Rough Chiton, Gumboot.

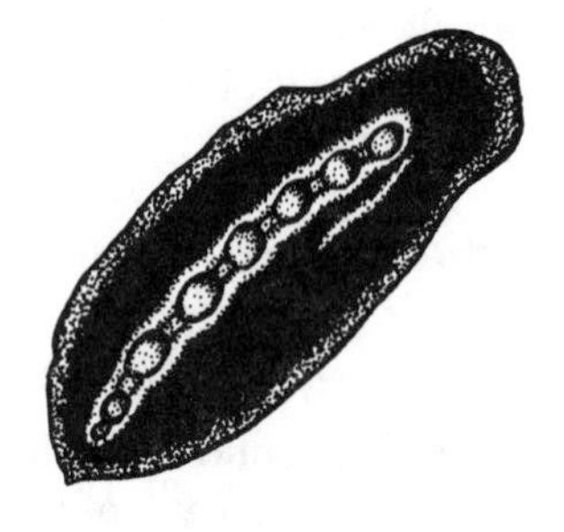

Black Turban Snail

Tegula funebralis

Shell to 1″ diameter, dark purple or black with four whorls. Ranges between low and high tide zones, feeds on algae. This is the most common snail on Pacific Coast. It can live to be 30 years old. Its shell is a favorite home for hermit crabs. Related species: Brown Turban Snail.

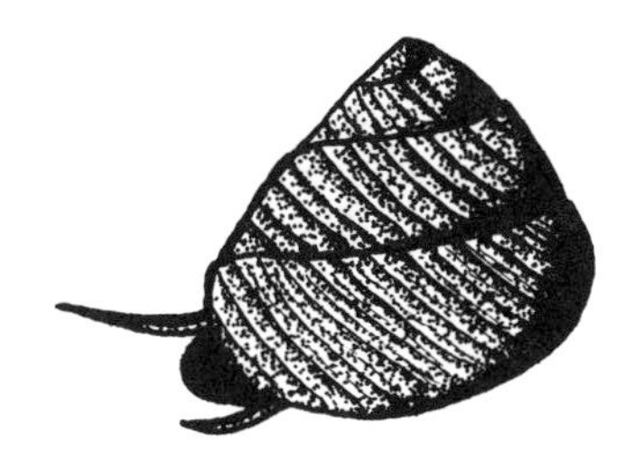

Acorn Barnacle

Balanus glandula

White, volcano-shaped shell to ¾″ wide. Often found in large colonies. Will attach to rocks, ships, shellfish, whales, etc. Eggs hatch into free-swimming larvae that eventually attach themselves permanently to a host. Barnacles eat plankton they strain from the water. Predators include sea stars, snails, worms, and certain fish and birds. Related species: Thatched Barnacle, Goose Barnacle.

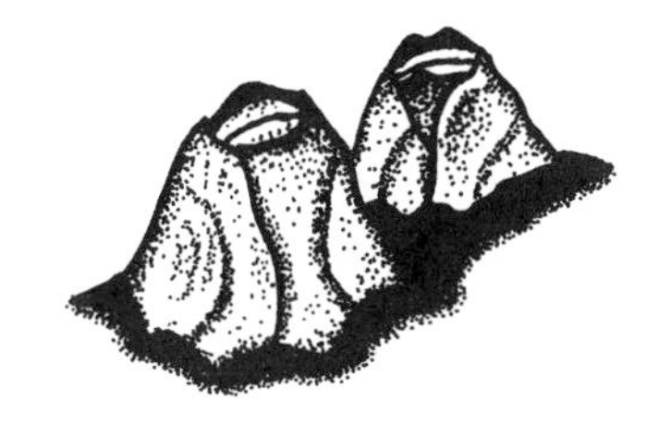

Bull Kelp

Nereocystis leutkeana

The most massive kelp of Northern California. Long, rope-like strands to over 100 feet in length grow from deep water. Strand ends in an elongated round air chamber that floats on the water's surface. Numerous flattened blades 10 to 12 feet long extend from the round bulb, hanging down into the water. After a storm, beaches may be covered with bull kelps torn loose and cast onto the shore. Despite their size, they complete their entire life cycle in a single year.

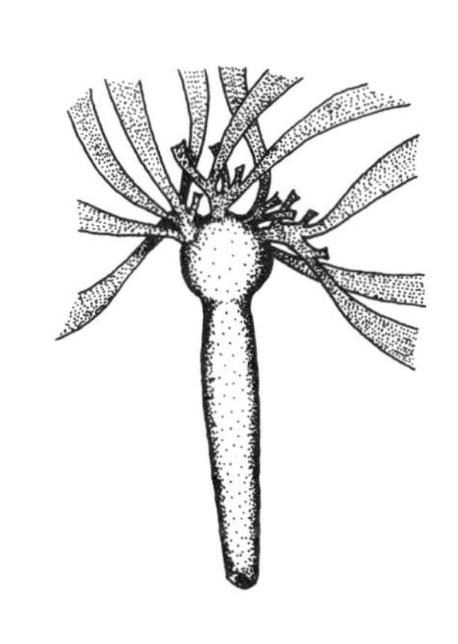

Red Sea Urchin

Strongylocentrotus franciscanus

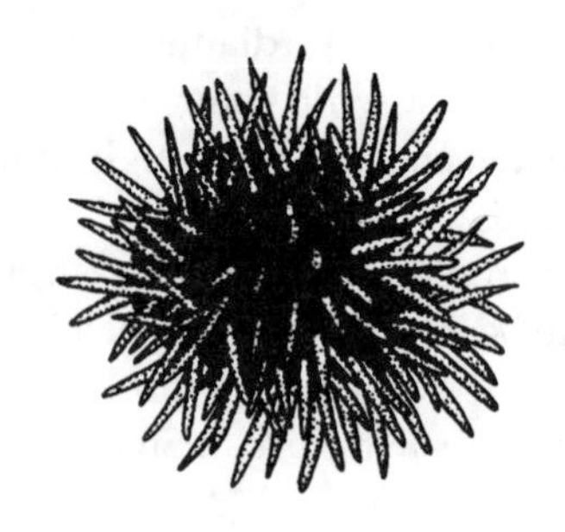

Spiny oval body to 5″ width with abundant spines up to 2½″ length. The fragile, shell-like body is formed of calcium carbonate. Spines are used for defense and for trapping algae. The urchin's mouth is a white, bony organ on its underside called Aristotle's Lantern. Urchins are a favorite food of sea otters, as well as sea stars, crabs, and man. Related species include the Green Urchin and Purple Urchin.

Ochre Star

Piaster ochraceous

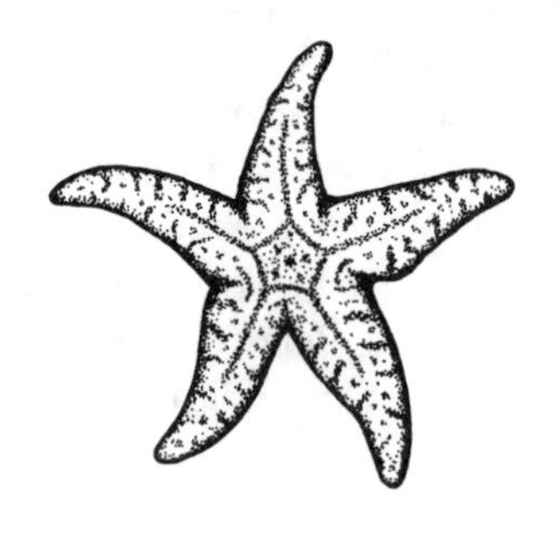

Can reach 10″ across. Yellow, orange, or reddish-brown body. This is the most common large sea star in tidepools and is often found in mussel beds. Like most sea stars, it can insert its stomach into a tiny gap in a mussel's shell to digest its victim. Sea stars are sometimes called "star fish," but this is incorrect because they are not fish. Related species include the Knobby Star and Leather Star.

Bat Star

Patiria miniata

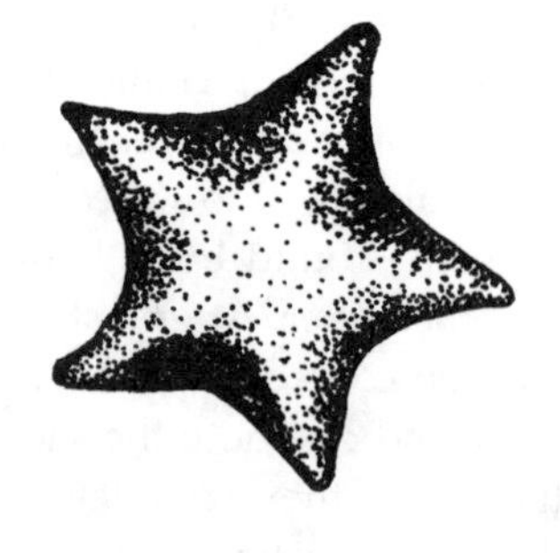

This small star can reach up to 4″ width. It is very common, especially in kelp beds. Color is variable, but commonly reddish-orange. It is found from the low tide zone to waters nearly 1000′ deep. Food includes other sea stars, sea squirts, and algae. Related sea stars include species with many arms: Sun Star, Sunflower Star, and Six-Rayed Star.

Daisy Brittle Star

Ophiopholis aculeata

Body diameter to 3/4″ with arms to 3″ length. Various colors, including orange, pink, yellow, white, blue, green, and black. These stars move rapidly when they are exposed by lifting away their rock cover in a tidepool. Several related brittle stars include the Dwarf Brittle Star, Western Spiny Brittle Star, and Burrowing Brittle Star.

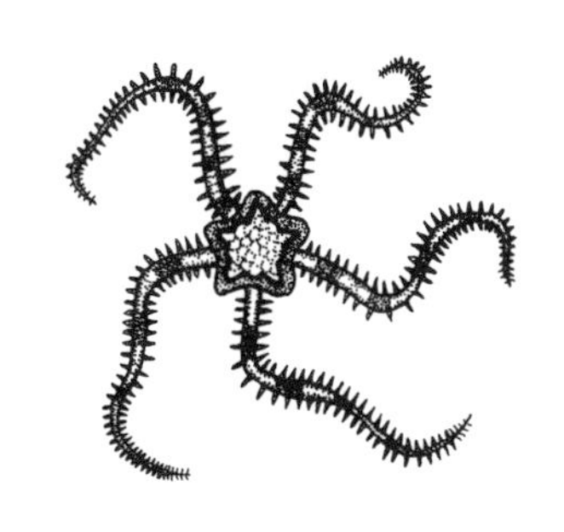

Purple Shore Crab

Hemigrapsus nudus

Deep purple body to 2¼″ width, 2″ length. Lighter colored pincers have many solid purple or red spots. Lives in rocky shores and seaweed from low to high tide zones. This common crab will quickly retreat into crevices when exposed. Several other species of crabs can be found in the tidal zone, including the Lined Shore Crab, Pacific Rock Crab, and Kelp Crab.

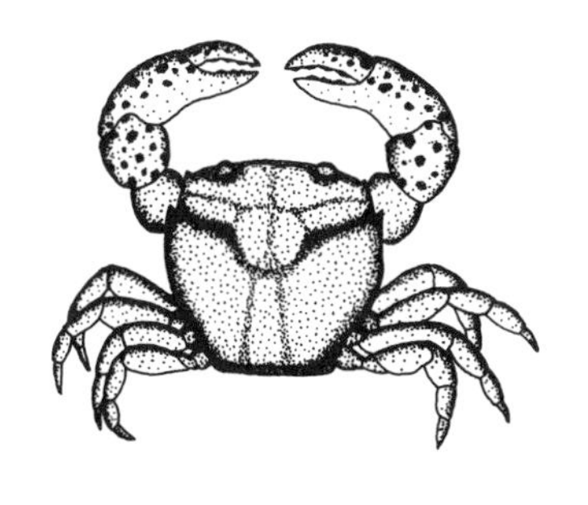

Blue-Banded Hermit Crab

Pagurus samuelis

Body reaches 3/4″ length, with blue bands on legs and pale blue pincer tips. Hermit crabs prefer shells of the black turban snail, and will frequently exchange a smaller shell for a larger one. These crabs are commonly found in the shallow waters of the mid and high tide zone. The related Grainy Hermit Crab is less tolerant of drying and so prefers the low tide zone.

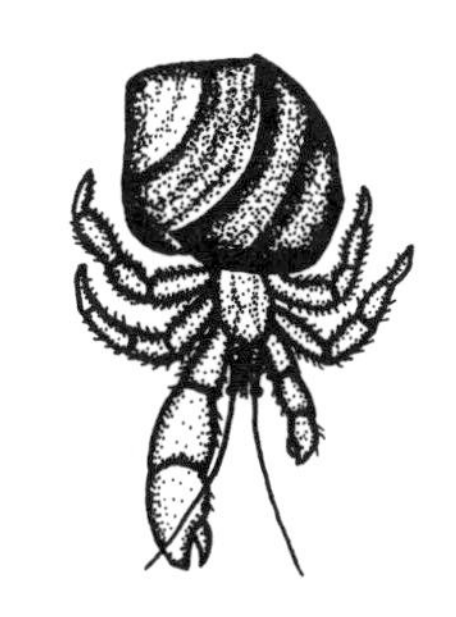

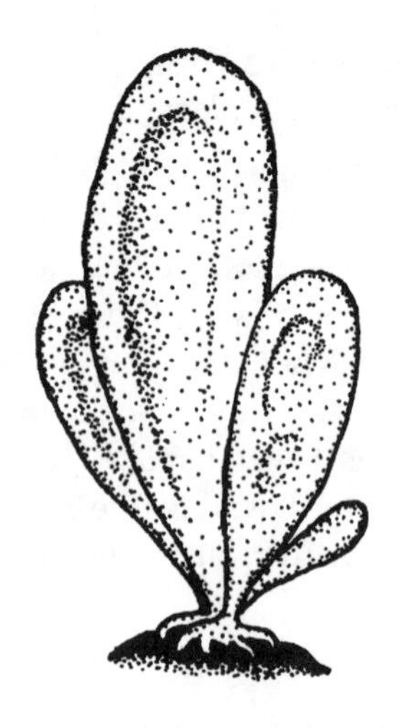

Sea Sack

Halosaccion glandiforme

Erect, water-filled sacks that can be up to 10″ long. Yellowish-brown in color. When squeezed, the sacks emit fine streams of water through several pores. Found in the mid tide zone.

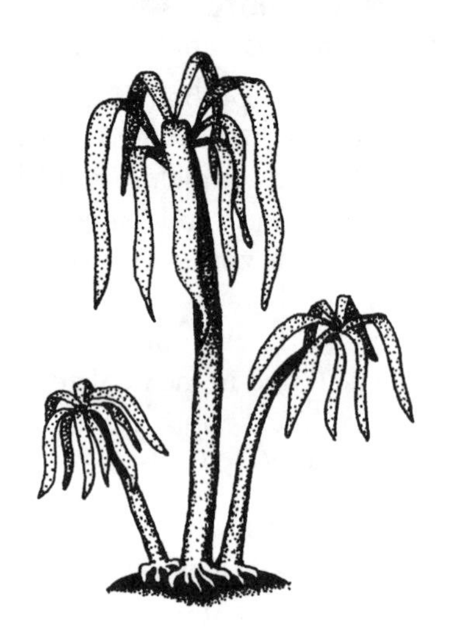

Sea Palm

Postelsia palmaeformis

Reaches heights to 2 feet. Dark greenish-brown in color. This aptly-named algae is reminiscent of a tropical palm tree. Often found in colonies clinging to rocks washed by strong surf. Best seen at low tide.

Appendix B

Common Marine Mammals of the Sonoma Coast

Pacific Gray Whale

Eschrichtius robustus

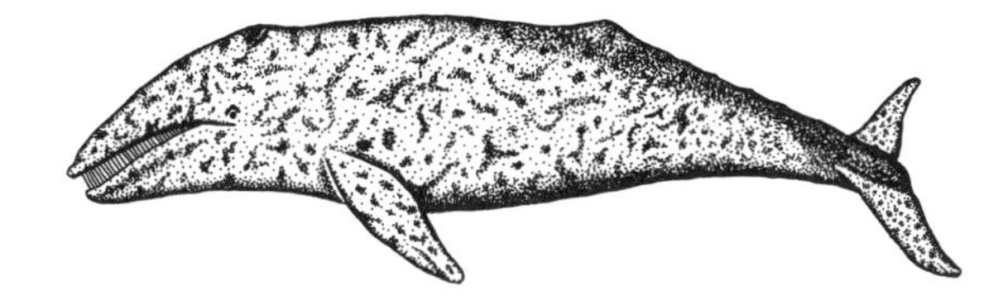

The Pacific gray whale is the most common whale seen off the Sonoma coast. Mature grays reach lengths of 40 to 45 feet and weigh between 17 and 35 tons. For whales, this is on the smaller side—the mighty blue whale, for instance, can reach 100 feet in length and weigh over 130 tons!

All whales are mammals, and they must come to the surface to breathe. Their nostrils, called blowholes, are located on the top of their head. To breathe, the whale normally thrusts only its blowhole above the surface. The spout of water you see when a whale breaks the surface is actually water vapor being expelled from its lungs as it exhales.

There are two types of whales: the *odontocetes*, or toothed whales, and the *mysticetes*, or baleen whales. The gray whale is a baleen whale and therefore has no teeth. Instead, it uses its baleen, a series of closely-spaced plates hanging from the roof of its mouth, as a kind of food strainer. Its primary food consists of amphipods—tiny shrimplike crustaceans that swim in great numbers in Arctic waters. (These amphipods are sometimes called "krill.") The gray whale feeds by rolling onto the sea floor and kicking up sediment containing amphipods. It then swallows a large quantity of this muddy water and forces it back out through the baleen. The mud and water are filtered out, leaving behind the amphipods to be swallowed.

Gray whales migrate annually from the cold Arctic to the warm waters of Baja California. The southern migration begins when the waters turn cold in October. Pregnant females depart first, for they must reach warm water before their calves are born. Next to leave are the non-pregnant females and mature males, followed by the juveniles. Courtship and mating are thought to take place along the migration path in early December. Gray whales tend to be solitary animals, so the migration occurs singly or in small groups, rather than in large herds.

Calves are born in the warm Baja waters the first two weeks in January after a 13-month gestation period. The northern migration begins in early February, starting with the females who became pregnant on the southerly journey. The males are next to leave, with the new mothers and calves bringing up the rear. It is believed that the whales do not feed during the entire migration and can lose one-third of their body weight by the time they return to their Arctic feeding grounds.

When watching for gray whales, it helps to have a vantage point above sea level. In Sonoma County, Bodega Head and Salt Point are two popular spots. You're more likely to be successful on days when the sea is calm and you can easily spot the whale's spout against the darker water. Don't discount overcast days, but windy afternoons when the sea is whipped with whitecaps are nearly hopeless.

The first thing you're likely to see is the spout briefly shooting above the water. This may occur close to shore or as far as several miles out to sea. A gray whale normally takes three to five shallow dives of less than a minute each, followed by a deep dive lasting over five minutes. You may see the whale's back gliding across the water as it takes a breath. Sometimes you'll see it lift its tail flukes above the water as it prepares to take a deep dive. On rare occasions you may even see a breach, where for some unknown reason the whale leaps entirely out of the water.

After being hunted for centuries and driven nearly to the point of extinction, the gray whale is today protected by international law. It is estimated that there are about 17,000 gray whales alive today, nearly back to its original numbers of 15,000 to 30,000 whales—a worldwide population still less than half the number of people living in rural west Sonoma County.

California Sea Lion

Zalophus californianus

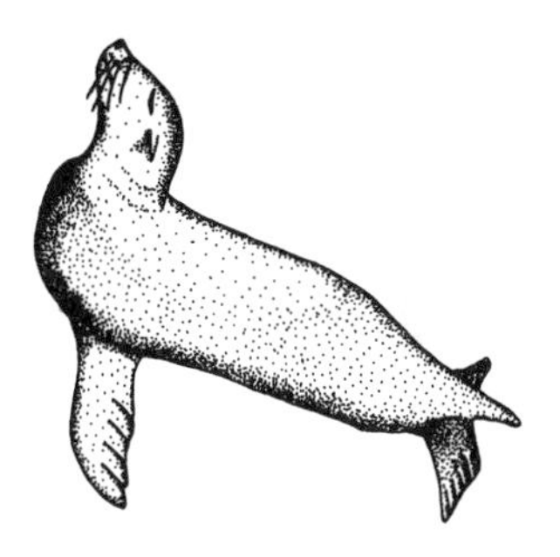

The trained seals you see in the circus are actually California sea lions. Males reach lengths of 6.5 to 8 feet and weights from 450 to 650 pounds. Females are much smaller, reaching lengths of 5 to 6.5 feet and weights of 100 to 200 pounds. They have noticeable external ears and their brown fur appears nearly black when wet. They gallop easily on land.

Sea lions are fast swimmers, reaching speeds up to 25 miles per hour. When swimming, they often "porpoise" through the water. They can stay submerged for up to 20 minutes and dive to 400-foot depths. Their diet consists of a variety of fish and mollusks.

Males are very territorial and will bark continuously when defending their territory. Mating occurs in June and July, with pups being born the following June. Sharks and killer whales are major predators. In past years sea lions were hunted for their blubber, but they are now protected by law.

Harbor Seal

Phoca vitulina

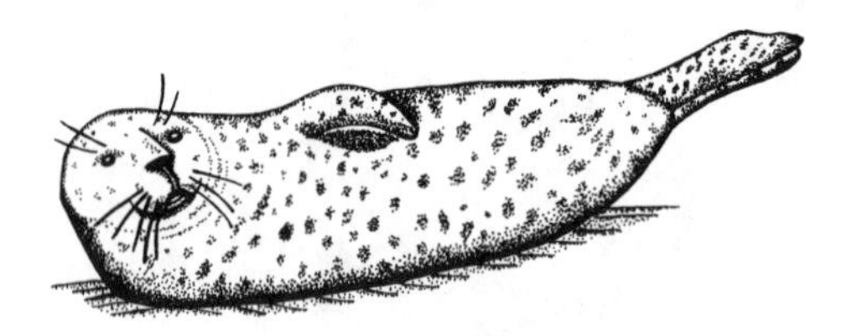

Harbor seals are a common sight along Sonoma County shores, often basking in large groups. They are somewhat smaller than sea lions and are distinguished by their yellow-gray spotted coat and by their lack of visible ears. They move clumsily on land solely by wriggling their bodies. When disturbed they raise their heads, then with an alarm bark they dive into the water. They can remain submerged nearly 30 minutes and reach depths of 300 feet.

The harbor seal's diet consists mostly of fish such as rockfish, herring, cod, mackerel and salmon. They feed at high tide, often swimming up rivers for their catch. As the tide recedes they haul out onto sandy beaches or rocky shores. Fishermen blame them for the large decrease in the salmon catch in recent times, though this is subject to dispute. For many years bounties were paid on harbor seals, but they are now protected by law.

The mating season varies by region, ranging from March to August. Males may breed with several females. They are hunted by killer whales, sharks, and in northern regions, by polar bears. Golden eagles have been known to prey on newborn pups.

Index

M

N

O

P

Q

R

S

About the Author

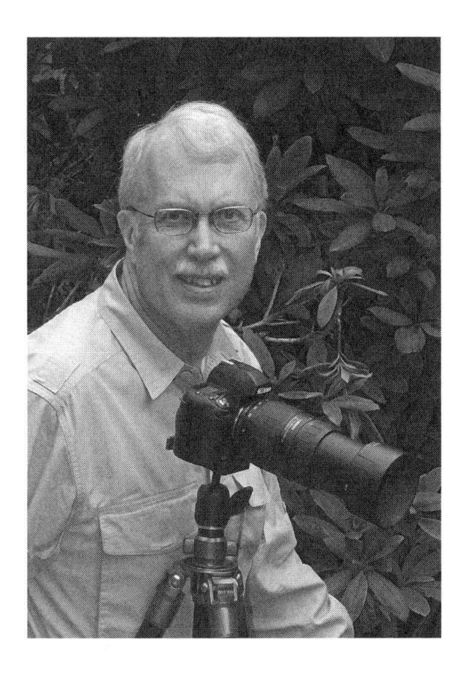

Steve Hinch has been exploring the Sonoma Coast since 1974. Born in Seattle, he grew up in the Southern California coastal city of Redondo Beach. His wilderness explorations began at a young age, when his avid rockhound parents would pack up the family and head out to remote desert locations in search of semi-precious stones nearly every weekend. He earned his way through college designing gold and silver jewelry for the family's custom jewelry store.

Trained as an electrical engineer, Steve has 30 years of management experience in the high-technology industry. He holds three patents and has authored three books. He is an expert on GPS navigation and is the author of ***Outdoor Navigation with GPS***, a bestselling guide to the subject for hikers, backpackers, hunters, mountain bikers, and other outdoor enthusiasts. Steve has two grown children and lives with his wife in the heart of the wine country in Santa Rosa, California. He is also an award-winning photographer who specializes in landscapes of the Southwest.

Stewards of the Coast and Redwoods

Stewards of the Coast and Redwoods (Stewards) is the non-profit volunteer organization that partners with the Russian River Sector of California State Parks to provide education and stewardship programs at Armstrong Redwoods State Natural Reserve, Austin Creek State Recreation Area, and Sonoma Coast State Park, including the Willow Creek watershed. Stewards also raises funds for resource management projects, and for assistance in the development of interpretive facilities. Their mission is to promote education, preservation and stewardship of the natural and cultural resources of Russian River area State Parks through interpretation and public stewardship. Over 350 volunteers contribute by providing park visitors of all ages with a variety of programs and opportunities to experience and explore these exceptional parks. In addition, Stewards routinely advocates for the needs of State Parks, ensuring they will be open and available for public enjoyment for generations to come. For more information or to join Stewards, please visit their website at www.stewardsofthecoastandredwoods.org.

Fort Ross Interpretive Association

The Fort Ross Interpretive Association (FRIA) is the California State Park Cooperating Association for Fort Ross State Historic Park and Salt Point State Park. FRIA is dedicated to the preservation, research, and interpretation of the cultural and natural history at Fort Ross and Salt Point State Parks. The Kashaya Pomo who have inhabited this area for centuries, the Russian-American settlement at Fort Ross in the early 19th century, and the pioneering American ranching and logging years which followed, are all part of this rich history. FRIA operates the Fort Ross Visitor Center and bookstore, maintains a library and archives, produces books and brochures about the cultural and natural history of Fort Ross and Salt Point, helps with the preservation of the fort, and sponsors cooperative projects and research with other organizations. For more information or to join FRIA, please visit their website at www.fortrossinterpretive.org.